WY

Resuscitation

For Churchill Livingstone:

Commissioning Editor: Ninette Premdas
Project Manager: Gail Murray
Project Development Manager: Valerie Burgess
Designer: George Ajayi

Resuscitation
A Guide for Nurses

Edited by

Annie Chellel BA (Hons) BSc (Hons) MA DipN RGN PGDE RNT
Senior Lecturer, Institute of Nursing and
Midwifery, University of Brighton, Sussex, UK

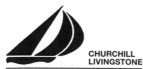

CHURCHILL
LIVINGSTONE

EDINBURGH LONDON NEW YORK PHILADELPHIA ST LOUIS SYDNEY TORONTO 2000

CHURCHILL LIVINGSTONE
An imprint of Harcourt Publishers Limited

© Harcourt Publishers Limited 2000

⬦ is a registered trademark of Harcourt Publishers Limited

First published 2000

ISBN 0 443 06187 4

British Library Cataloguing in Publication Data
A catalogue record for this book is available from the British Library

Library of Congress Cataloging in Publication Data
A catalog record for this book is available from the Library of
Congress

Note
Medical knowledge is constantly changing. As new information
becomes available, changes in treatment, procedures, equipment and
the use of drugs become necessary. The editor, contributors and the
publishers have, as far as it is possible, taken care to ensure that the
information given in this text is accurate and up to date. However,
readers are strongly advised to confirm that the information,
especially with regard to drug usage, complies with the latest
legislation and standards of practice.

Printed in China

Contents

Contributors

Sue Adams MSc RN SCM RCNT CertEd DipNurs(Lon)
Senior Lecturer and Course Leader MA in Nursing, Institute of Nursing
and Midwifery, University of Brighton, Sussex, UK

Ruth Austin BSc(Hons) RGN ENB 100
Resuscitation Training Officer, Princess Anne Hospital,
Southampton, UK

Jane Cant BSc MA
Clinical Risk Manager, Southampton University Hospitals NHS Trust,
Southampton, UK

Shiona Gardiner Barrister at Law BSc LLM RGN RSCN RNT
Barrister at Law, Maidstone, UK

Caz Holmes BSc RGN RSCN ENB 415 APLS Instructor
Paediatric Resuscitation Training Officer, Guy's and St Thomas's NHS Trust,
London, UK

Barbara Plumb RGN ALS Instructor PALS Provider Resuscitation Council
(UK) PHTLS Provider Royal College of Sugeons England
Resuscitation Officer, Kent and Sussex Weald NHS Trust, Pembury
Hospital, Tunbridge Wells, UK

Steve Rochester ALS PALS Instructor FETC
Resuscitation Officer, ALS and PALS Instructor, Resuscitation
Council (UK), Eastbourne District General Hospital, Eastbourne,
UK

Diane P. Smith BSc(Hons) EN RGN DPSN CertEd RNT
Senior Lecturer, Institute of Nursing and Midwifery, University of
Brighton, Sussex, UK

Alison Snow RGN CertEd ENB 254
Resuscitation Training Department, Princess Anne Hospital,
Southampton, UK

Brian John Stone MSc DipRespMed
Resuscitation Officer, The Conquest Hospital, Hastings, UK

Michael Ward BS MB FRCA
Consultant Anaesthetist, Nuffield Department of Anaesthetics, The John
Radcliffe Hospital, Oxford; Past Chairman, Resuscitation Council, UK

Clive Weston FRCP
Consultant Cardiologist, Department of Cardiology, Singleton Hospital,
Swansea, UK

Preface

I remember vividly the first resuscitation attempt I saw as a student nurse: I was shocked by the noise, the drama, the urgency and the brutality. I recall my fear and my emotional distress, and my grim reflections on the fragility and value of human life. It was my fear of not knowing what to do in the event of a cardiopulmonary arrest that led me to do an intensive care course soon after I qualified, with the intention of returning to surgical nursing. Once I had acquired the knowledge and skills to cope, my fear dissolved; I began to enjoy the challenge and the excitement of trying to save a life. I loved the one-to-one ratio of intensive care, where I have remained for 20 years. During that time I have been involved in many, many resuscitation attempts in intensive care and on occasion in other wards, departments, corridors, lifts and car parks. This book is intended to help nurses understand their diverse role in resuscitation attempts and to provide the knowledge they need to take part without fear in the team effort. It is my hope that it will offer support to nurses, whatever their specialty, by exploring the issues that are relevant to their unique contribution and perspective.

Emergency situations, such as resuscitation attempts, test the structural systems, equipment, resources and working practices of the National Health Service as well as the skills, knowledge, experience and teamwork of those, like nurses, who work within it. A successful outcome in resuscitation is, of course, a surviving patient, since that is the purpose of the endeavour. The structure and process must be considered successful, however, if all the necessary equipment, drugs and personnel were immediately available and worked together in a coordinated, well organized and scientifically based resuscitation attempt. We can and should be proud of that achievement because we can be confident that everything possible was done to save a life. If death ensues, it is the inevitable result of some underlying trauma or pathology rather than inadequacy on the part of the Health Service. Many people are involved in the constant testing, teaching and rehearsal that are necessary to ensure that call systems, equipment, drugs and skilled personnel are immediately available at all times.

In recent years the quality of resuscitation attempts has been greatly improved by the work of the Resuscitation Council (UK), which has standardized and simplified the management and teaching of cardiopulmonary resuscitation. Standardized multiprofessional courses in resuscitation are excellent at providing participants with basic life support skills and knowledge of the algorithms and their rationales for advanced life support. They are practised and tested in the safety of artificial scenarios using mannequins and some Oscar-winning performances by teachers and students. This preparation for practice is, of necessity, achieved by teaching resuscitation as a mechanistic process with little time for discussion of its human impact or research findings, which indicate very low survival rates. As I am a nurse, this raises ethical issues and professional dilemmas for me which I need to address. The nursing perspective – which includes spiritual, emotional and caring factors – makes resuscitation a more complex, demanding and prolonged event for nurses. This book was inspired by the need to articulate that perspective.

Nurses must understand the nature, extent and purpose of their roles and responsibilities in resuscitation so that they can accept their professional accountability to patients and colleagues. These may vary according to the nature of their daily practice, but all nurses may be called upon to resuscitate at any time and in any context. Their role in the team effort to save a life goes beyond the immediate physical requirements of the arrested patient. Nurses have an important role to play before (in the case of patients they have nursed), during and after resuscitation attempts.

Nurses are able to acquire knowledge of the individual patient through nursing assessment and the creation of a trusting and caring nurse–patient relationship. This allows nurses to learn important details about the patient's expectations, beliefs and wishes. Such knowledge is essential if the patient's rights and dignity are to be respected as death approaches. Ethical and legal dilemmas can be resolved more easily if the patient's own voice is heard, and it is usually a nurse who is there to listen and record what they have to say about their care. Resuscitation attempts on unconscious and unknown individuals are more difficult because we do not know their history, their prognosis or their wishes about whom they want to be informed or what they would want us to do for them.

The nursing role during resuscitation requires scientific knowledge about cardiopulmonary arrest, its aetiology, signs, symptoms and treatment. It is also concerned with the human impact of this life-threatening event on all who are involved. The spiritual and emotional consequences of death or near death may affect inexperienced staff, relatives, other patients or the surviving patient. Supporting shocked, frightened and grieving people demands time and attention at a moment when the immediate physical needs of the resuscitation attempt must take priority. This inherent conflict of need is a mirror of the more fundamental conflict for nurses between the peaceful and dignified death we would wish for our patients, and the violence and intrusion of resuscitative interventions.

When the resuscitation attempt ends nurses have to deal with its consequences. This may involve the transfer of a surviving patient to a hospital or to an intensive care unit, or it may involve dealing with the death of a patient. Nurses may have to inform and comfort relatives and support inexperienced staff. Nurses often have to clear away used equipment and ensure that it is cleaned or replaced, ready to be used again. The other nursing responsibilities of the shift must be taken up again and witnesses to the event will need to be given support.

This book aims to support nurses in this complex role. The first section (Chapters 1 to 5) which begins with a brief history of resuscitation and the Resuscitation Council (UK), is concerned with issues relating to the art of nursing. Legal and ethical aspects as well as the care of relatives are explored. The role of the nurse is discussed, integrating the related nursing theory with decision making in practice. Spiritual aspects and the caring role of the nurse in resuscitation are included, and the near death experience is examined through some of the related research and literature.

The second section, Chapters 6 to 13, is concerned with the scientific knowledge nurses require as the foundation for their practice in resuscitation. The guidelines from the European Resuscitation Council (1998) form the basis of this section. The algorithms of basic and advanced life support are explained including the drugs used, and there are chapters on defibrillation, and airway management. Paediatric and trauma life support are included from the nursing perspective and there is a chapter on resuscitation in the community. The research on outcomes is reviewed to provide a more realistic view of the chances of survival than is indicated by television dramas!

Obviously a book on resuscitation is no substitute for its practice, and it is strongly recommended that readers should ensure that they update their skills by undertaking practical courses. This book offers a theoretical supplement to nurses undertaking such courses but also provides the necessary knowledge base for nursing practice in resuscitation.

Resuscitation is a wide and expanding subject and this is reflected in the varying backgrounds of those who have written chapters according to their particular interest in this field. I am very grateful to the authors and it is a tribute to their commitment to this subject that they have somehow managed to find time for writing between the demands of a full day's work and family life. I believe that our efforts have produced an interesting book which nurses will find informative and useful.

Anne Chellel

Tunbridge Wells 2000   Annie Chellel

Resuscitation: past, present and future?

Michael Ward

INTRODUCTION

Imagine for a moment that you are unfortunate enough to suffer a cardiac arrest in the mid-eighteenth century. The chances are, that your friends and relatives would offer up a prayer of thanks to the Almighty for your life but little more would have been done as the idea of resuscitation from cardiac arrest was entirely unknown. That, of course, assumes that you were not arresting as a result of having fallen into a river or the sea. The 're-animation' of the apparently dead, withdrawn from water, appears to have been actively pursued and a number of the techniques then in use are well described in the literature. If you were really lucky, you would have been thrown across the back of a horse and trotted along, head down, for some time. If you were unlucky, and the facilities had been available, smoke from burning wood chips would have been insufflated into your rectum! The rationale for the former, viewed through modern eyes, appears quite acceptable. The head-down posture would have helped drain water from the lungs, and the trotting produced rhythmical compression of the chest against the horse's back which may have both aided respiration and produced a certain amount of cardiac compression to provide an artificial circulation. The rationale for the second technique seems lost in antiquity. Perhaps it was the act of passing the insufflator per rectum that bought about stimulation but the only stimulation now that would be recognized by such a manoeuvre would have been vagal slowing, which would be unlikely to assist restart an hypoxic myocardium.

EARLY ATTEMPTS AT RESUSCITATION

In the mid-eighteenth century, the first organization that attempted to provide a system of care for the near drowned victim was set up in

Amsterdam (1767). In 1774, the London Society for the Recovery of Persons Apparently Drowned was established, under the direction of Drs William Hawes and Thomas Cogan (Bishop 1974). This organization changed its name in 1776 to become the Humane Society and in 1787 came under royal patronage. Rewards were given for the delivery of bodies found in the London stretches of the River Thames, to designated depots where resuscitation equipment was available. Such equipment included the ventilating bellows and mouth-to-nose ventilating apparatus. Unfortunately, there is little record of the success rate of these organizations.

The Humane Society reported on matters other than resuscitation from drowning, and in their Proceedings for 1775 is a description of successful electrical defibrillation (Julian 1975). This was performed at University College Hospital in 1775 on 3-year-old Sophia Greenhill, who fell out of an upper storey window, and was said to be 'to all appearance dead'. She was taken to the Middlesex Hospital where it was declared that nothing could be done for the child. A Mr Squires tried the effects of electricity – 20 min elapsed before he could apply the shock, which he gave to various parts of the body in vain. However, upon transmitting a few shocks through the thorax, he perceived a small pulsation; in a few minutes, the child began to breathe with great difficulty, and after some time she vomited. A kind of stupor, occasioned by the depression of the cranium, remained for several days but, by the proper means being used, 'her health was restored'. It is difficult to explain the outcome but the case generated so much interest in the use of electricity that many other references to its use appear in the subsequent reports of the Humane Society. Regrettably, few details of the method of electrical therapy are given.

In 1819, Giovanni Aldini, nephew of Galvani, published his studies on 'The Application of Galvanism for Medical Purposes, Particularly in Cases of Suspended Animation'. However, the use of electricity was severely limited by the means of generating it, since the devices that were available at the time were large and extremely cumbersome.

By the mid-nineteenth century, devices for the provision of respiratory support were being widely described and numerous techniques were developed to achieve 'artificial respiration'. This was still largely in the area of resuscitation from drowning but was occasionally applied to victims of other forms of sudden death. Artificial ventilation provided by these external means continued in popular use until the mid-twentieth century when, in 1946, James Elam described the use of mouth to nose, expired air ventilation. He collaborated with Peter Safar to develop the concept of mouth-to-mouth ventilation (Safar 1958).

The first documented use of external cardiac compression occurred in Germany in 1891, when Friedrich Maass, a surgical assistant to Professor Franz Koenig of Göttingen, adapted Koenig's technique for artificial respiration to produce a pulse in two patients suffering from cardiac arrest during chloroform anaesthesia (Taw & Maass 1991). However, the use of such closed chest massage did not catch on, for a number of reasons. It must be remembered that myocardial infarction, today's commonest cause of unexpected cardiac arrest, was not a recognized disease, only being described as such since 1912. Most physicians rarely saw patients with unanticipated arrest and the majority of patients who did arrest, did so during anaesthesia with chloroform and generally responded to ventilation. Where arrest was unresponsive in this surgical environment, the logical approach was to use direct internal massage of the heart to stimulate a response and to produce an output. The unavailability of a practical method to defibrillate also rendered the technique superfluous. Thus, the concept of external chest compression that had been described was not widely known or practised.

THE BEGINNINGS OF MODERN RESUSCITATION

In Johns Hopkins University, Baltimore, MD, USA, in the mid-1950s, while studying the effect of various manoeuvres on dogs with fibrillating hearts, Jude, Kouwenhoven and Knickerbocker realized the efficacy of production of an artificial circulation by the application of pressure to the closed chests of dogs. They studied the effect of various positions, pressures and rates and eventually applied the technique to humans, publishing their findings in 1960 including the sentence 'Anyone, anywhere, can now initiate cardiac resuscitative procedures. All they need is two hands' (Kouwenhoven et al. 1960).

It was now possible easily to combine the twin elements to produce an artificial circulation and artificial respiration. The combination became recognized as cardiopulmonary resuscitation (CPR) and the mnemonic 'A, B and C' was popularized to remind practitioners of the essential elements: Airway, Breathing and Circulation. The American Heart Association led the process by endorsing the technique and setting up a CPR Committee. Together with the US National Research Council of the National Academy of Science and the American Red Cross, they convened an ad hoc conference that published the first standards for training and performance in CPR (Ad Hoc Committee on Cardiopulmonary Resuscitation of the Division of Medical Sciences, National Academy of Sciences–National Research Council 1966).

Improvements in modern resuscitation techniques coincided with a better understanding of the electrophysiology of acute cardiac death. Much of this work was stimulated by the increasing use of domestic electrical power and the increasing incidence of electric shock induced ventricular fibrillation. Indeed, much of Kouvenhoven's early research (Safar 1989) was funded by grants from the New York Edison Power Company. For a long time electrical defibrillation was referred to as 'countershock'.

Claude Beck, Professor of Surgery in Cleveland, OH, USA, was the first to develop and use a defibrillator in humans. His first successful case was a 14-year-old boy undergoing surgery for severe funnel chest who suffered a cardiac arrest as the chest was closed. Beck reopened the chest and directly massaged the heart for 45 min until his newly developed defibrillator was available in the operating theatre. Two shocks, applied directly to the open myocardium, were required before the heart returned to sinus rhythm.

Three hours later, the boy was sufficiently recovered both from his ether anaesthetic and his 45 min of 'death' to answer questions. He made a full neurological recovery (Beck et al. 1947). Beck also recognized the fact that sudden cardiac death from coronary artery disease was not necessarily due to cardiac necrosis, but to acute rhythm disturbance and coined the much quoted phrase 'hearts too good to die'.

It was another 8 years before external defibrillation was tried successfully in humans. As an extension to his pioneering work on cardiac pacemakers, Paul Zoll developed a device designed to apply an AC charge through the chest wall. He published his findings in 1956 when he had successfully stopped ventricular fibrillation 11 times in four different patients, but with only one survivor (Zoll et al. 1956). One of the greatest obstacles to further development was that alternating current devices required a mains source of AC and a step up transformer, which prevented portability and limited availability. Bernard Lown (Lown et al. 1962) solved that problem when he realized that a DC shock could be equally effective and replaced mains power by battery and eliminated the transformer. The new DC defibrillator, while originally neither lightweight nor easily portable, at least permitted it to be quickly transported to the patient either in or out of hospital.

Once it was appreciated that resuscitation could be successfully achieved in patients suffering sudden cardiac arrest, it became apparent that there was a need for rapid provision of CPR until definitive treatment such as defibrillation was available. With this recognition that resuscitation had to be started promptly after collapse, attention was turned to the provision of aid in the community. Frank Pantridge, with the aid of a grant from the British Heart Foundation, established the world's first mobile coronary care unit (MCCU) in Belfast in 1966. Staffed by an ambulance driver, physician and nurse its aim was to reach rapidly, patients with a diagnosis of acute myocardial infarction so that they could be present in the event that ventricular fibrillation occurred. Their early work (Pantridge & Geddes 1967) covered 312 patients over 15 months during which there were 10 cardiac arrests, all of whom were admitted to hospital and five were discharged alive.

MODERN RESUSCITATION

Since those early days, the concept of pre-hospital provision of CPR and advanced life support (ALS) has grown. All UK ambulances now carry a light, portable defibrillator and a trained paramedic. However, the success of treatment for cardiac arrest in the community still depends on early intervention, often by a bystander. The British Association for Immediate Care set up a Public Liaison Committee in 1980, following suggestions by Asmund Laerdal that the public awareness in the provision of basic life support (BLS) needed to be increased. This group was chaired by Judith Fisher, a general practitioner in East London, UK.

The Public Liaison Committee underwent a total reorganization and rebirth in 1981 following the granting of financial support from the British

Heart Foundation, to become the Community Resuscitation Advisory Council (CRAC). Its aims were to review resuscitation standards, such as there were, and to give advice to the community at large in the UK on all aspects of resuscitation. In addition to its Chairman, its seven inaugural members are well known to modern students of resuscitation – Peter Baskett, Douglas Chamberlain, Rodney Herbert, Andrew Marsden, Mark Harris, John McNee and David Zideman. CRAC, in cooperation with the voluntary organizations, the St John Ambulance and British Red Cross produced a number of booklets and leaflets with flow charts to aid in the teaching and performance of BLS by members of the lay public.

Over the next few years, it became clear that not only the lay public required further information regarding resuscitation. In 1984, the Community Resuscitation Advisory Council reinvented itself as the Resuscitation Council for the United Kingdom, a registered charity with four major objectives:

- Public education in life-saving skills
- Education of doctors, nurses, ambulance personnel and other health workers in all aspects of resuscitation
- To investigate and encourage research into all areas of resuscitation
- To disseminate the useful results of such research to as wide an audience as possible.

Membership of the new Resuscitation Council was by invitation and was offered to medical practitioners who demonstrated a continuing interest in resuscitation matters. It began to issue early guidance to the medical profession but it was not universally popular, partly because its studies began to show that existing medical practices were not based on sound scientific principles. Indeed, it was described by one group of its opponents as a 'self-appointed group with no standing'.

Some centres were already beginning to recognize the time-consuming, but essential value of good-quality resuscitation training. The Royal Sussex Hospital, Brighton, UK, appointed a dedicated resuscitation trainer in the person of Mr 'Dusty' Miller who had previously been employed as an ambulance technician. His post was soon to be copied and it is likely that the first nurse to occupy a dedicated resuscitation training role in the United Kingdom was Geralyn Wynn at the Royal Free Hospital London.

In 1986, the Resuscitation Council (UK) was still the only group of medical practitioners dedicated to the pursuit of excellence in resuscitation matters and, as such, it was invited to play a major part in the BBC television 'Save a Life Campaign' of that year. The campaign was run under the joint auspices of the Royal Society of Medicine, St John Ambulance, Red Cross and the Resuscitation Council (UK). With the enthusiastic support of the BBC, the campaign had as its objective the training of in excess of 1 million members of the public in BLS. It has been calculated that its 20-min television programmes giving instruction to the public were seen by in the region of 50% of the adult population of the UK. At the close of the campaign in 1987 it was able to claim that several lives were saved directly as a result of members of the public following the lessons they had learned from the television programmes and attending the supporting resuscitation training sessions.

Tom Evans, consultant cardiologist at the Royal Free Hospital was then invited by the British Medical Journal to edit a series of articles on resuscitation matters for their ABC series. He asked his colleagues on the Council to contribute and the first edition proved to be so popular it has been updated and republished as new editions in 1991, 1995 and 1999. In the 1980s, resuscitation was becoming a recognized speciality interest area but, unfortunately, it was still not being carried out or taught within hospitals in any controlled or systematic fashion. A working party of the Royal College of Physicians published a report in 1987 entitled 'Resuscitation from Cardio-pulmonary Arrest: Training and Organization'. The Report recommended the establishment of specialized training staff to be responsible for the training of all hospital personnel in a systematic resuscitation system that would be reproducible and practical. These new resuscitation training officers were beginning to be appointed in centres of excellence and the Royal College of Physicians' report encouraged their appointment even within district general hospitals. The other main recommendation of the report was that the organization and control of resuscitation should be under the direction of a resuscitation committee to be chaired by an interested anaesthetist or physician.

The British Heart Foundation (BHF) agreed to make a major contribution towards the funds required by hospitals to create new posts and this resulted in an enormous boost to the establishment of resuscitation training officers. The BHF grants were for half the required funding for up to 3 years, provided that the employing hospital agreed to take over the funding subsequently. Applicants for such posts came from a number of occupations, but were principally nurses with a critical care interest.

With the increasing popularity of resuscitation skill acquisition, the Resuscitation Council (UK) was becoming larger and a special general meeting in 1988 looked at its future and agreed five important points for development. These were:

- The Council should continue to consist only of registered medical practitioners
- These should be elected after submission of a CV and be nominated and seconded by existing members of Council
- The setting up of a council executive limited to 20 persons to manage the Council
- The establishment of a Finance and General Purposes Committee to manage the day to day running
- A number of working groups would be set up with the power to co-opt personnel from outside the Council whose role was to develop guidelines and encourage research in their special areas.

The working groups of the Council at that time were set at six: BLS, ALS, paediatric life support, near-drowning/hypothermia, research and training.

At that time similar, but less well developed, groups were also beginning to appear in other European countries. An informal meeting of interested individuals was held during the European Society of Cardiology Annual Meeting of 1985 and proposed the setting up of a working group of that Society, to concern itself with resuscitation matters. The proposal received the approval of the council of the Society and was put to the general assembly at Dusseldorf in 1986 but was rejected. (The feeling at that time was that resuscitation was not a cardiologist's issue.) As a result of this rejection, this same group of cardiology enthusiasts who recognized the need for the development of a European multidisciplinary body, set up a meeting in Antwerp in 1988, chaired by Douglas Chamberlain but organized by Leo Bossaert: thus was born the European Resuscitation Council.

The Resuscitation Council (UK) continued with its charitable aims to improve the education of medical and paramedical staff by holding regular annual symposia. The first of these was held in the Hammersmith Hospital, London, UK, in 1990 and has been held there every year since. The first European Congress of the European Resuscitation Council was held in Brighton, UK, in 1992 hosted by the Resuscitation Council (UK). It was opened by Her Royal Highness, The Princess Royal and this helped to achieve some publicity in the general media, thereby advancing the discipline of resuscitation in the UK. Other aims of the Resuscitation Council (UK) were achieved in 1992 by the publication of the BRESUS Study (Tunstall-Pedoe et al. 1992), a survey of 3765 cardiopulmonary resuscitations in British hospitals and which is now regarded as the datum point for resuscitation.

The Council was then still very much at 'cottage industry' status and had largely operated out of the department of anaesthetics, Hammersmith Hospital. It was then recognized that the Council activity would grow with its plans to initiate a structured ALS course and it was felt necessary to look for its own premises. In 1993, the Council moved into 9 Fitzroy Square, London, to occupy part of the building owned by the British Cardiac Society and appointed a course coordinator to run the increasingly popular ALS course. With the increasing expansion of the activities of the Council it was soon found necessary to appoint a general administrator and the Council was fortunate to appoint Fiona Whimster, who was seconded to work with the Council from her post as coordinator of Bart's City Life Savers. By 1997, in addition to the administrator, there were six full-time employees and it became increasingly necessary to look for larger accommodation. The Council moved to BMA House in Tavistock Square, London.

The main reasons for the expanding activities of the Council are success with its courses for medical and paramedical personnel. These include the ALS, the paediatric ALS and the instructors courses. It is also anticipated that a newborn ALS course will commence in 2000. The Council is increasingly referred to by the public, the profession and the media for views on resuscitation matters and has taken the opportunity to publish reports on areas of general interest. These include the publication on whether relatives should be present during resuscitation and guidelines for anaphylaxis. Future publications will also cover community resuscitation, resuscitation equipment and advisory external defibrillation. The other aim of the Council, that of encouraging research (largely by the provision of seed-corn funding), is actively pursued, with financial backing and encouragement given to a number of studies throughout the UK. Examples of projects that have received support are the study of the risk of defibrillation in the presence of glyceryl trinitrate (GTN) transdermal patches, the development of new techniques of minimally invasive internal cardiac massage and the ongoing audit of resuscitation practice in the UK.

NEW INITIATIVES AND TRAINING

The Resuscitation Council (UK) is actively involved within Europe and was invited by the national societies of both Italy and Portugal to assist with the development of their own *ad hoc* ALS courses. Members of the UK Council are chairs, or co-chairs of all the subcommittees of the ERC and were instrumental in guiding the development of the International Liaison Committee on Resuscitation (ILCOR). ILCOR's recommendations for resuscitation were published in 1997 and adopted (or will be adopted within 3 years) by the UK, the rest of Europe, Australia, Southern Africa and South America. It is expected that they will be accepted by North America in the new millennium. These new guidelines are the result of international consensus with rationalization of existing national guidelines using scientific evidence, where this is available. It is hoped that once all national groups follow the same protocols, training and research will be globally applicable and acceptable, with savings of time and effort and, hopefully, a reduction in mortality. When global guidelines are achieved, international standards can be set and opportunities for research on a multicentre, multinational basis will be enhanced.

Training in ALS in the UK is now almost entirely under the aegis of the Resuscitation Council (UK) whose ALS manual appeared in a third edition in 1998, following the European Resuscitation Council's Congress formal acceptance of new guidelines. The ALS course is controlled by a subcommittee of the Council consisting of medical, educational and resuscitation training officer representatives and courses must follow a common core content and programme, which together with faculty must be approved by the Council. The $2\frac{1}{2}$-day course includes didactic lectures, practical and role-playing sessions. Successful completion of the course provides a certificate that is valid for 3 years. Acute specialities and areas are increasingly making possession of a valid ALS certificate a key requirement for employment.

Good performances on an ALS course, combined with good leadership and training potential can be identified by the course faculty and suitable candidates may be put forward as 'Instructor Potential' (IP). Such IP providers are encouraged to assist on provider courses and then advance by attending an instructors course. This 2-day course is run in selected centres using the skills of experienced trainers and educators and aims to encourage best practice in adult education techniques.

The UK's ALS course is successful and is being acquired by the ERC for translation into many European languages, although it may require adaptation to meet local needs and practices. With its acceptance by a greater European community comes increasing opportunity for mobility of personnel and research. Greater cooperation with the North Americans is essential, so that the American Heart Association advanced cardiac life support (ACLS) course is not regarded as competition with wastage of resources. Eventual harmonization under the aegis of the respected ILCOR should be the aim.

CONCLUSION

The future of resuscitation rests on the validation of our current practices, concepts and beliefs through active research, especially large multicentre investigations of structure, process and outcome. However, such research can be valid only if all resuscitation attempts follow the standardized guidelines.

The foundation will be that of a sound scientific basis for standardized and practical guidelines that will ensure better outcomes for those who could, and should, survive cardiopulmonary arrest. The Resuscitation Council (UK) is dedicated to this work nationally, the European Resuscitation Council internationally within Europe and, in the future, one hopes to see ILCOR develop into a group able to look globally.

REFERENCES

Beck C S, Pritchard W H, Feil H S 1947 Ventricular fibrillation of long duration abolished by electrical countershock. Journal of the American Medical Association 135:985–986
Bishop P J 1974 A short history of the Royal Humane Society to mark its 200th Anniversary. Royal Humane Society, London
Cardiopulmonary Resuscitation Committee on CPR of the Division of Medical Sciences, National Academy of Sciences–National Research Council 1966 Cardiopulmonary resuscitation: a statement by the Ad Hoc Committee on Cardiopulmonary Resuscitation of the Division of Medical Sciences, National Academy of Sciences–National Research Council. Journal of the American Medical Association 198:138–145, 372–379
ILCOR 1997 Advisory statements for resuscitation. Resuscitation 34(2):99–150
Julian D G 1975 Cardiac resuscitation in the eighteenth century. Heart and Lung 4:46
Kouwenhoven W B, Jude J R, Knickerbocker G G 1960 Closed chest cardiac massage. Journal of the American Medical Association 173:94–97
Lown B, Amarasingham R, Newman J 1962 new methods for terminating cardiac arrhythmias; use of synchronized capacitor discharge. Journal of the American Medical Association 182:548–555
Pantridge J F, Geddes J S 1967 A mobile intensive care unit in the management of myocardial infarction. Lancet ii:271–273
Resuscitation Council (UK) 1998 Advanced life support provider manual, 3rd edn. Resuscitation Council (UK), London

Royal College of Physicians 1987 Resuscitation from cardio-pulmonary arrest: training and organization. Journal of the Royal College of Physicians of London 21(3)

Safar P 1958 Ventilatory efficacy of mouth-to-mouth artificial ventilation. Journal of the American Medical Association 167:335–341

Safar P 1989 History of cardiopulmonary–cerebral resuscitation. In: Kaye W, Bircher N (eds) Cardiopulmonary resuscitation. Churchill Livingstone, New York, ch 1

Taw R L Jr, Maass F 1991 100th anniversary of 'new' CPR. Clinical Cardiology 1:1000–1002

Tunstall-Pedoe H, Bailey L, Chamberlain D, Marsden A, Ward M, Zideman D 1992 Survey of 3765 cardiopulmonary resuscitations in British hospitals (the BRESUS study). British Medical Journal 304:1347–1351

Zoll P M, Linenthal A J, Gibson W *et al*. 1956 Termination of ventricular fibrillation in man by externally applied electrical countershock. New England Journal of Medicine 254:727–732

FURTHER READING

Eisenberg M S 1996 The quest to reverse sudden death: a history of cardiopulmonary resuscitation. Chapter 1 In: Paradis N, Halperin H R, Nowak R M (eds) Cardiac arrest – the science and practice of resuscitation medicine. Williams and Wilkins, Baltimore, 1–27

Ethical aspects of resuscitation

Jane Cant

2.

■ CONTENTS

INTRODUCTION

Involvement in any resuscitation attempt, be it successful or not, inevitably brings with it a heightened sense of professional and personal anxiety and disquiet. That disquiet is significant. In dramatic moments such as resuscitation, by virtue of your actions, you are compelled to express your moral responsibilities as a nurse and your ethical reasoning as an individual. Difficulties arise when certain values, beliefs or moral principles collide. Moral reasoning will help you in your decision-making when faced with the complex ethical dilemmas, which cast their shadow over so many resuscitation attempts.

This chapter aims to provide a framework for more critical deliberation than may be customary. I do not pretend to provide you with the answers: ethical reasoning is a process not a product and the unique nature of each patient and their situation requires individual consideration. However, what I can offer is the opportunity to use a framework to inform your decision-making. Throughout this chapter, I have posed questions (indicated by bullet points) that you need to consider in order to assist in clarifying your thoughts and feelings about the ethical issues of resuscitation in your clinical environment. Finally, it may be helpful for you to remember that your ability to accept moral responsibility and the quality of your ethical reasoning will be a measure of your professional competence.

WHAT ARE THE ISSUES?

Ethical insecurity and conflict may be inherent in any resuscitation situation. You may have the luxury of time and be able to discuss how to proceed in the event of a patient arresting. Deliberate pre-emptive discussion, which involves the patient in the decision about their own resuscitation, is a clinical treasure. All too often, however, resuscitation attempts are sudden, without warning, and the resulting action has to be immediate, deliberate and very physical. There are no half measures. This raises many questions for nurses:

- How do you feel about it?
- Do you have a process for decision-making?
- What is it that bothers you?
- How do you resolve any differences that you encounter within yourself or with your professional colleagues?
- Have the patient's wishes been made known to you?

To illustrate, accompany me on an ethical 'ward round' (Case history 2.1), then you can ask yourself whether your reasoning is based on personal prejudices or pure philosophical persuasions.

Case history 2.1

William Scott is 74. He is brought into the Accident and Emergency (A&E) department having collapsed at home with sudden chest pain radiating up his neck and jaw. He is overweight and has been a heavy smoker for 35 years. He is identified as being hypertensive and cardiovascularly unstable. He arrests as he is being examined.

Deborah is 22 years old and in the past year has been admitted to hospital 14 times following a bone-marrow transplant. She is readmitted with a chest infection and renal failure. Her condition continues to deteriorate and, in the opinion of the staff, there is little hope. Deborah has a 3-year-old son and her own parents are keen that all resuscitative measures are taken. She has a cardiac and respiratory arrest before a definitive decision has been reached.

John King is 63 years old and has chronic obstructive pulmonary disease (COPD). Over the last few years he has been progressively house-bound with significantly deteriorating pulmonary function. He has been admitted previously and spent 3 weeks in the intensive care unit (ICU). His family is a large and supportive one, and includes a number of grandchildren. His consultant believes that there is little chance of him being weaned off the ventilator should his condition worsen. Mr King is keen to return home, even if he were to be ventilator dependent.

A 75-year-old male is brought into the A&E department, having been found unconscious in his flat. A neighbour had become concerned and had rung the emergency services. Beside the man was a neatly written note stating that as a widower for 6 years he no longer wished to live. An empty bottle of tricyclic antidepressants was found at his home. He arrests as he is moved onto a stretcher.

Maureen Frampton is 48 years old and recovering in the cardiothoracic ICU following an aortic valve replacement. Postoperatively, she has recurrent problems with ventricular tachycardia/fibrillation. This continuing sequence of events responds well to DC shocks but continues during the afternoon. Her husband, continuously at her bedside, becomes instrumental in alerting the attending staff to the impending dysrhythmias. Over 2 h later, the staff feel the situation is not improving and they wish to withhold treatment. Her husband, however, is adamant that treatment should continue.

While names have been changed, the cases are all real ones and there are, of course, many more.

- What were your first reactions?
- Were you guided by intuition or a 'gut reaction'?
- Did you take time to consider the alternatives?
- If Mr Scott arrests, would there be some prejudices that get in the way?
- How many times have you been in a situation where the 'Deborahs' of our experience have left you feeling confused and distressed?
- What considerations would you have to take into account when deciding what would be the best course of action for Mr King?
- How would you deal with the dilemma of the deliberate suicide attempt and the possible anger should he survive?
- What do you see are the boundaries for relative participation and their presence at cardiac arrests?
- What principles do you use in discussing and negotiating the withdrawal/withholding of treatment?
- Who decides?

Ethical issues lie at the centre of the difficulties many nurses experience when involved in resuscitation attempts. It will frequently be you at the bedside initiating that crucial response. Equally, it will frequently be you who is at the bedside when a do not resuscitate (DNR) order is sanctioned. Effective cardiopulmonary resuscitation can be life sustaining; without it, death is inevitable. In order to feel empowered to initiate crucial ethical debates you must have some understanding of the moral theories and principles that shape our world.

COMPETING MORAL THEORIES

There is an underlying assumption that medical ethics is inextricably bound and justified by fundamental moral theories (Gillon 1992). The two major theories belong to deontology and consequentialism. I offer simple explanations of both, but you should be aware that simplification for the sake of brevity carries the risk of distorting these complex philosophical arguments.

Deontological theories espouse individual obligations and obedience to certain moral rules. It is the behavioural action as a moral duty that is essential, not the outcome or consequence of that action. Many deontological theories, such as those espoused by Immanuel Kant (Kant 1948), rely on the principle of absolutism. You may well believe that we are morally obligated to tell the truth, or never do any body any harm.

- Should Deborah have been told that should she arrest little hope existed that she would survive?
- Would that have led to 'harm' by increasing her anxiety and distress?

Where one fundamental and absolute moral principle collides with another, logical argument could result in constraining us from acting correctly. The acceptance of moral pluralism and a desire to find a resolution between competing moral principles has led to differing deontological approaches. Moral obligations may be seen as those duties we would intuitively accept, such as duties and obligations that involve truth-telling, doing good, not harming others, duties of gratitude and justice and compensation, and also those more recently expressed under the tenets of Clinical Governance, namely duties of life-long learning, self-improvement and professional self-regulation. Rawls (1976) believes that there are opportunities to rank these conflicting principles in order of priority: while other philosophers believe that resolution comes from discussion of opinions rather than from absolute knowledge. It is a dispute in itself that cannot easily be settled.

Within the ethical dilemma of a resuscitation attempt:

- What is your standpoint?
- Is it at odds with the views of the patient or with any of your clinical colleagues?
- Do you believe that in some specific circumstances, certain moral principles are applied to determine a resolution?

Consequentialism, however, justifies the rightness or wrongness of actions according to the outcome: maximizing the greatest good for the greatest number is the basis of all utilitarian ethical theories. Bentham (1968), a proponent of utilitarianism, claims that it is a moral theory based on the principle of maximizing welfare. Happiness and suffering, for example, are not conflicting principles but are at opposite ends of a continuum. Since there are no competing principles, decision-making is based on identifying the course that will produce the most happiness or least suffering:

- What would you decide in the treatment of Mr King?
- With his hugely supportive family and his desire to watch his grand-children grow up, what might be the decision based on the theory of utilitarianism?

Difficult philosophical problems arise:

- What is meant by happiness?
- How does one measure it?
- How can happiness be maximized and how would one calculate total happiness?

Considering the scope of happiness:

- Does the philosophical framework encompass all things, animals and humans alike?
- How does it deal with the unborn, the very young or the permanently unconscious?

While these concerns are not restricted solely to utilitarianism, there are clear counterintuitive concerns. If we review the ordinary moral deontological principles that inform the way we develop relationships (such as respect for each other's autonomy, for truth-telling, integrity, openness, honesty, fairness and justice), utilitarianism would expect us to ignore some or all of these principles in the overall maximization of happiness and societal welfare.

Contemporary teaching of ethical theories supports the view that the consideration of rights, based moral philosophy, should sit alongside deontology and consequentialism. There is no doubt that the language of today is heavily charged with moral claims of individual rights, often requiring either action or restraint in dealing with others. Gillon (1992) considers the distribution between legal and institutional rights and those that are defined as moral rights. Legal and institutional rights are those that are created (or abolished) by parliament or social institutions, such as the right to free health care and education. The new Patient's Charter espouses the rights of individuals to health care provision. In addition a revised Health Bill (DoH 1999) not only imposes a statutory duty of care with service provision, but now a statutory duty of quality is imposed, to support the government's new 'National Health Service and the Clinical Governance' initiative.

John Locke, a seventeenth-century physician and philosopher promoted the theory of God-given moral rights of man. Within the context of medical ethics, one fundamental human right exceeds all others, that of autonomy (the right to exercise one's freedom through self-determination by consent or by refusal). It is a right that often imposes a reciprocal obligation or duty on others. Within the health-care setting, we see claims made to the universal moral right of life, particularly in the context of resuscitation. An individual's claim to the right to life may impose upon others an obligation that feels wrong or implausible.

- Do you believe in a universal right to life such that there must be a reciprocal moral obligation to keep that person alive?
- Do you consider this a universal moral right and one that is absolute? If not, what are the moral demands and the extent of your professional obligations?
- Is there discordance within the context of any defined resuscitation setting?
- How could a DNR decision fit within this moral philosophy?

It is true that this language of human rights may be extended to the consideration of the moral duties of others. We have a duty, not only to respect autonomy, but to respect another's dignity, to do good, to do no harm and to seek justice and fairness. Equally, within this philosophical paradigm, each one of us has a moral right to decide for ourselves, to defend our own freedom and to protect our personal autonomy. The tensions, I hope, are becoming all too obvious.

PROFESSIONAL OBLIGATIONS

It is worth remembering that medical ethics have been guided by moral rules and declarations that go back as far as the Hippocratic oath. The duties owed to Mr Scott, Deborah and John King, for example, are identified through adherence to such principles as honesty, confidentiality, informed consent affirming the patient's right to privacy, dying in dignity, maintaining respect for human life and relieving suffering. Such codes of medical practice are found in the Declaration of Helsinki (1964) (BMA 1993), the Declaration of Lisbon (1981) (Gillon 1992), the Declaration of Tokyo (1975) (BMA 1993) and the Declaration of Venice (1983) (Gillon 1992). As nurses, certain principles are embodied within the UKCC (1992) Code of Professional Conduct and in the UKCC's publication *Guidelines for Professional Practice* (UKCC 1996). Consider the range of both duties and rights expressed in the following excerpt:

'As a registered nurse, midwife or health visitor, you are personally accountable for your practice and in the exercise of your professional accountability must:
1. Act always in such a manner as to promote and safeguard the interests and well being of patients and clients.
2. Ensure that no action or omission on your part or within your sphere of responsibility, is detrimental to the interests, condition or safety of patients and clients.
3. Maintain and improve your professional knowledge and competence.
4. Acknowledge any limitations in your knowledge and competence and decline any duties or responsibilities unless able to perform them in a safe and skilled manner.'

If it has been a long time since you examined the contents of these documents, I recommend that you find your copies and read them again. The difference this time will be that you are now able to start analysing the inevitable moral conflicts between individual rights and reciprocal duties that make up some of your ethical dilemmas.

More recently, within the tenets of Clinical Governance, professional duties of accountability, self-regulation, life-long learning and efforts to ensure the highest possible standards echo key moral principles. It is important to ask yourself questions such as:

• Is my knowledge base up to date?
• How competent am I in dealing with an arrest situation?

- Do I regularly ensure I am clinically competent in resuscitation skills?
- Is the information that I give to patients and their relatives honest and accurate?

It should now be clear to you that many of your professional obligations are rooted in fundamental moral principles and these may have a direct impact on situations of cardiac/respiratory arrest and resuscitation decisions. Since our lives are framed within the context of a pluralistic society, rights and duties are often in conflict and therein lie the ethical dilemmas that nurses so frequently face in their daily practice.

APPEALING TO ORIGINAL PRINCIPLES

Individuals often lay claim to an original ethical principle to justify their position. Such principles are those of autonomy, beneficence, nonmaleficence and justice. I will briefly review these principles in the context of resuscitation but further reading is recommended (Beauchamp and Childress 1983).

Autonomy

Autonomy is the right of an individual to be self-governing. As a principle, it advocates self-determination and relies on an individual having the capacity to think, decide and act on the basis of such thoughts, and to make decisions freely and independently (Gillon 1992). Within the clinical context, it demands that individuals ought to have liberty to decide how to live their lives and, indeed, to be able to exercise control over their life and death plans. Inevitable questions arise:

- How applicable should this principle be?
- Does it apply to all human beings in all situations?
- Should the autonomy of Deborah or Mr King be respected, irrespective of the costs incurred?
- Should the patient who had deliberately taken an overdose be resuscitated or be allowed to die?

Let us first examine this situation. If we use Kant's deontological perspective, Kant believed that one must never treat any individual as a means to an end. In addition, in exercising one's autonomy, the principle must conform to the requirement of rationality. Actions are considered right if the motivation is derived from the universal principle of autonomy based in rationality. For Kant, suicide is wrong because it adopts the contrary principle of making use of the person as a means rather than as an end. It would also be questionable that, since the decision was not considered rational according to universal laws, it could not be considered as autonomous. Similarly, in applying the utilitarian principle of maximizing happiness, assurance to the public that all efforts to protect the sanctity of life in emergencies must be protected.

The decision to resuscitate also appeals to the principle of beneficence in conflict with that of non-maleficence. This conflict of principles is one commonly seen within the context of advance directives. While in the first instance advance directives appeal to the principle of autonomy, we frequently use Kant's argument of irrationality. Frequently the Kantian principle of respect for the autonomy of another individual might be ignored if incomplete information has been given and/or considered by that individual.

Situations involving information giving and informed consent are founded on the principle of autonomy. It is no easy matter to determine what and how much information constitutes 'enough'. If the individual is not sufficiently informed then that person's autonomy is automatically impaired. Similarly, if information is presented in such a way that might influence choice, then autonomy is limited.

- Is it your experience that in all situations, patients are given appropriate information in order to decide for themselves whether they wish to be resuscitated in the event of an arrest?
- If not, why not?
- Should Deborah or Mr King have been involved in pre-emptive discussions about resuscitation?

As a consequentialist, your approach might be different. Remember that autonomy is only to be valued if it yields the best outcomes. You may believe that in some situations the best outcomes are achieved when incomplete or biased information is given. The individual then chooses that treatment regarded by the clinical team as being the most appropriate.

- In your experience, how often does this happen?
- How comfortable do you feel about it?

Autonomy and paternalism

It is often the conflict between autonomy and paternalism that leads to much discomfort. The recognition of autonomy has enormous intrinsic value in the relationships we have with others. Inherent to such relationships are honesty, confidence and truthfulness.

- Do you believe that there are any clinical situations that justify paternalistic interventions by clinicians?

The major resource unavailable to you in an arrest situation is time. Split-second decisions that you have to make are often immutable. The pressure to make such decisions in intense situations when the patient lacks decision-making capacity has a tendency to make practice paternalistic. Frequently, immediate unilateral decisions have to be made about saving a person's life. Lack of time prohibits collaborative discussion. In other situations, your own values and the patient's ability to exercise their own autonomy may be in direct conflict. Justification often comes in the form of an argument in favour of reducing the patient's anxiety – an appeal made in the name of both beneficence and non-maleficence.

- Do you agree that such an appeal legitimizes a less than honest approach, false confidence, evasions, deceit and paternalistic decision-making?
- How often do you give your patients an opportunity to decide for themselves if they would wish to be resuscitated?

Initiating such open and honest debate with the patients for whom you are caring would minimize paternalistic practice and optimize autonomous choices (see chapter 3 on legal issues and chapter 4 on the nurse's role in resuscitation attempts). It is ironic that in situations where patients may be deceived and expectations falsely supported – in the name of their best interests – it is often the relatives that are told the truth, and thus duplicity in the deception is propagated. However, it is possible that some patients really do wish to be shielded from unpleasant information and have decisions made for them. Nursing skill lies in the investment of time and effort for the assessment of patients, in order to find out just what they really want. The danger is that paternalistic assumptions, by definition, undermine the principle of autonomy.

It is certainly true that we find it awkward discussing with patients their wishes in the event of an arrest and explaining the likely consequences, good or bad. It is, however, much harder to make and come to terms with decisions when we really have no idea what the patient would have wanted. Arguments that individuals are not capable of understanding medical terminology or the implications of treatment decisions are now strongly refuted. With the development of individual rights, the growth of health-care consumerism, increased access to medical information and the concept of active participation in treatment decisions, paternalism is now increasingly regarded as unethical behaviour. Solutions to ethical problems are not the sole prerogative of health care professionals. Instead, solutions rely on participation of the team and, most importantly, the individual whose life and death is affected by the decisions that have to be made.

Beneficence and non-maleficence

The principle of beneficence promotes the concept that well-being or benefit of the individual ought to be promoted. Conversely, non-maleficence promotes the principle that one must do another no harm (Singleton & McLaren 1995). As a consequentialist, the two principles may be seen to be at opposite ends of the same continuum. Treatments are designed to provide overall benefit to the individual, thus, while there may be some pain and suffering involved, generally the individual patient benefits. In a resuscitation attempt, despite the physical pain, indignity and intrusion of supportive measures, the benefit of life tips the balance in favour of active measures. In evaluating the rightness and wrongness of our actions, it is the consequence of those actions that is important.

Deontological supporters, like Kant, view the principles of beneficence and non-maleficence as being significantly distinct. The latter principle applies to everyone as a 'perfect duty', meaning that there is no exception: each one of us has a duty not to harm anyone else. Beneficence, however, is an 'imperfect duty': that is, that we do not have a duty to benefit everyone. There is an element of latitude in deciding whom one should help.

- Within your own clinical practice, does this distinction fit with your common sense intuition?
- What do you consider to be the range or limitation of the principles of beneficence and non-maleficence?
- How is it possible to assess benefits and harms especially in the situation of resuscitation?
- What is counted as well being or harm?
- Whose concept of these terms is being used: is it your own, is it one shared by the health care team, is it that of the individual who is the subject of these decisions?

Conflicts arise since these terms are often individually defined. The death of a patient may be viewed as the ultimate harm, while for others it may be seen as a benefit in bringing release from suffering and a lingering death. It is an argument that could well be used in the care of Mrs Frampton. Ideally, what is needed is the individual's own assessment of what these alternatives may mean. It is clear that benefits and harms need to be weighed against each other. It is also clear that individual conclusions may vary significantly as to what well-being means to each of us. In our example, Mr King expressed a wish that, whatever the ensuing consequences, the overall benefit would be to spend time with his family.

- Should that decision be overridden?
- Given that Mr King's decision is, in addition, an autonomous one, how would you justify advocating for a different outcome?

Research and resuscitation

- What is your knowledge of research findings in the field of resuscitation?
- What are the issues involved that makes this a hugely contentious area?

The pursuit of knowledge is embodied within the discipline of research. The guiding principle of medical research is autonomy, but it is influenced by the principles of beneficence, non-maleficence and justice. The welfare of the patient must be respected as primary and superior to the values of science, social and self-interest. Access to human subjects for research is a sensitive privilege, which any investigator is duty bound to respect. Equally, human experimentation is a necessity if new treatments are to be discovered and validated. Regulatory measures, such as the Declaration of Helsinki (1964, revised 1975), have done much to place essential constraints on human research. The Declaration requires, among other things, that the researcher should obtain the subject's freely given informed consent. In resuscitation situations where prior consent is not commonly obtainable, opportunities to research new treatment regimens are almost automatically precluded. It is an immensely difficult problem, both ethically and scientifically. The safe rule has always been that the possible loss of knowledge cannot outweigh the possibility of harm to the subject, even if the utilitarian calculation indicates great benefit to many and harm to only a few.

- How then, can research, which seeks to maximize resuscitation survival, be constructed as being ethically responsible?
- If a different family of drugs is suspected as being equally effective in resuscitation, how can such clinical investigations be framed?

Any compromise might endanger patients and abuse the privilege of human research (Monagle & Thomasma 1994). Without research, resuscitation is in jeopardy of becoming a marginalized area of emergency health care. It is a difficult conundrum.

Justice

The principle of justice, attributed to Aristotle, is that equals should be treated equally: with it comes the requirement that individuals should be equally considered, with fairness and impartiality. According to Gillon (1992) this complexity and diversity in the theories of justice prevents a 'generally acceptable substantive position'. The reason for such varied responses is largely due to the differing relative weights individuals place on the moral principles of autonomy, beneficence and non-maleficence. The questions you must ask yourself include:

- Which principle most protects people's individual rights?
- How is welfare best maximized?
- If I believe in the principle 'each according to their need', how would I define 'need'?
- Should medical resources be allocated according to individual merit rather than illness?

Distributive justice and the allocation of scarce medical resources are thorny issues. A consequentialist approach to both the macro- and micro-allocation of healthcare resources may be judged by the overall benefit achieved. But how do we measure benefit? Williams (1992) has suggested that benefit can be measured according to units of a quality adjusted life year (QALY). This approach, favoured by economists, also has its critics. Health means different things to different people. The quality of life measures used in the development of the QALY were based on limited criteria so that generalizability is questionable. Moral arguments focus on the consequentialist calculations of benefits.

- Do you believe that distributive justice should have overall outcome as its central tenet, where individual lives are of secondary importance?
- Do you hold more deontological principles, similar to Rawls (1976), primarily respecting individuals as ends in their own right?
- Is randomization the only equitable approach to resource allocations and access to treatment (Harris 1985)?

- What decision would you make in the case of Mr Scott or Deborah?
- What are the prevailing ethical principles you would appeal to in making your decision?

Perhaps, at the very least, justice is about giving due consideration to the competing ethical principles and identifying which fundamental moral value is to be given priority. After all, as Gillon (1992) proposes, 'justice is precisely a method for moral resolution of conflicting claims'.

MEDICAL FUTILITY AND DO NOT RESUSCITATE ORDERS

If we are accepting that it is not appropriate to resuscitate all patients, difficulties often arise in explaining what may be 'instinctive' decisions not to resuscitate. Instigating a do not resuscitate (DNR) order is in direct conflict with the moral imperative of the right to life. However, as has been asked before, is it life at any cost and does that right always imply a reciprocal duty to resuscitate? It is clearly not so, as seen in the context of any DNR order. Therefore, what ethical principles are appealed to in making such decisions?

- Do you initiate discussions about withholding or withdrawing treatment?
- Do you feel obliged to initiate resuscitation attempts you know to be inappropriate?

Since consent or refusal lies at the root of self-determination, the most preferred option must be to ask the patient. There are problems, but in circumstances where there are opportunities to do so, you must discuss those options. Patient assessment should include asking the patient about their wishes regarding resuscitation and whom they would like to be informed first. This information should be recorded in the patient's nursing notes and communicated to those involved in their care. It is also true that successful resuscitation varies according to the setting or patient group. Equally, its success is frequently overestimated by both health professionals and probably more so by the general public. It would appear that discussion between patients and their carer regarding resuscitation is the exception rather than the rule. Discussions between patients and health-care professionals need to be honest and timely. Knowing what the patient wishes would pre-empt many an ethical struggle.

- What if the patient wishes to be resuscitated even if the outcome is likely to be poor or render the individual severely disabled?
- Do patients have a right to what might be considered as a useless intervention?
- What is meant by 'medical futility'?
- Are we in jeopardy of confusing futility arguments with economics?
- Is futility part of the wider debate about rationing?
- How comfortable are you with the concept of futility?

It is worthwhile at this point to examine briefly what might be meant by the term 'futility'. Withholding cardiopulmonary resuscitation (CPR) from patients, based on the argument that it is futile therapy, is likely to have profound implications ethically, medico-legally and financially. So what is 'futility'? It might be useful to restrict the definition of futility to a medical determination rather than a patient's own conclusion. It has already been identified that a patient has the right to refuse therapies that he or she considers futile, morally objectionable or disproportionately burdensome, with or without the concurrence of his or her clinician.

Medical futility, then, is a medical determination that a therapy is of no value or benefit to a patient and therefore should not be prescribed. The current and contentious debate hinges around whether this constitutes an unacceptable form of medical paternalism or whether the concept of 'medical futility' provides for an appropriate clinical approach based ultimately on the beneficence model. I do not in any way wish to impugn medical motives, but wish to emphasize that close scrutiny in situations such as withholding treatment or providing life-sustaining measures is required.

Miles (1994) has identified the following four clinical types of futility:

- therapies that are physiologically implausible
- therapies which are considered 'non-beneficial'
- therapies which are very unlikely to produce a desired physiological or personal benefit
- therapies that have not been validated (although may appear plausible).

Problems still remain in defining the meaning of 'non-beneficial'. The question still to be asked must be, 'Non-beneficial (and therefore futile) in relation to what?'

Do you consider 'futility' solely in terms of death or survival? Or do you consider the probability of outcome in qualitative terms? Put into context, how should futile CPR be defined? And at what point might the decision be made that a treatment is futile? How would you deal with a situation where a patient considered that a very small chance of survival on life-support following CPR was beneficial? In your experience, if a medical decision of futility has been made regarding CPR, are patients informed as to the do not resuscitate (DNR) order? In your view, does a decision not to use medically futile therapy devalue life?

There are obvious tensions between the concepts of medical futility, autonomy and justice. What is also clear is that a deeper understanding of the term futility at the very least provides a framework within which these contentious issues can and should be explored and perhaps reconciled.

Clearly, there are bound to be emergency resuscitation situations where the principle of patient autonomy cannot be exercised. The implications of who decides what, is profoundly difficult. It is clear that a DNR order should not come from a unilateral declaration of futility. It is a decision that must emerge from collaborative discussion. Current debates about medical futility remain both contentious and important. You might believe that withholding treatment on the basis of futility is an unacceptable expression of medical paternalism. Conversely, you might believe that DNR decisions are made according to sound clinical calculations and that the burdens of treatment will outweigh its benefits.

- How would you define futility?
- Is this the case with Mrs Frampton?
- It might be so, according to your clinical judgement, but what ethical argument would you use?
- Can you see a difference, if you are appealing to the principle of beneficence or non-maleficence or even justice?
- If you believe that life should not be prolonged at all costs, what circumstances might justify decisions that would inevitably lead to the death of a patient?
- You have to ask yourself the question – what is the meaning of life?
- Does 'life' equate to the way in which we live our lives, our social interactions, personal relationships, happiness and fulfilment?
- Does 'life' imply having some ability to function at a cognitive level?
- What do you understand by the term 'person' or 'personhood' and how might it affect your decision-making?

These are huge ethical issues that need to be explored in much more detail in order to understand your personal beliefs and prejudices. What do words such as futility, life and personhood mean to you?

As you can see, there is an ethical and clinical fragility about invoking the term 'futility', but it can provide a framework within which the value of life is respected and where professional responsibility, the inevitability of death, beneficence, non-maleficence and even justice can be reconciled. Indeed, the issue has been given national recognition with the publication of a joint statement from the BMA and RCN in association with the Resuscitation Council (1993), which outlines specifically when a DNR decision may be appropriate. It is not surprising, however, that many of the fundamental ethical issues raised within the statement remain open to conflicting interpretation.

CONCLUSION

Throughout this chapter, I have referred to principles of honesty, truthfulness, trust, respect, patient dignity and confidentiality. These are all essential prerequisites for a successful patient–clinician relationship, but they are values that are all too easily undermined. Resuscitation can be shocking: shocking in its indignity, in its sheer 'physicality', its violence and often in its aftermath. It is inevitable that as a nurse, you care about your patients and are affected by these experiences. This is entirely as it should be, for to be untouched by a resuscitation attempt would be fruitless indeed. Caring is quintessential to your professional practice (see chapter 4), but it comes at a price. Recognition must be made that a restorative period is needed for all staff involved in resuscitation attempts. For nurses, perhaps more than for others, the situation does not suddenly go away. Continuing high-dependency care for the patient who survives, transfer to the ICU and care of the deceased and their relatives remain high priorities for nursing staff. The effect can be traumatic and distressing. Frequently, insufficient consideration is given to the staff involved, to the stress they experience and to how they may be feeling after this dramatic event.

- Did the resuscitation go according to plan?
- Are there lessons to be learned?
- Were the right decisions made?
- Who made the decisions and how were they made?
- Did everyone agree?

Whatever the clinical decision, meticulous record keeping and documentation are essential for both the medical and nursing professions.

Ironically, it is frequently the case that areas which have a proportionally greater number of arrests, spend less time in ensuring that staff feel well-supported in the aftermath. The next patient may be waiting to be admitted, yet nurses sense the indignity of the haste to move on. You must recognize those human needs and values both in yourself and in your colleagues. If you are in a position to be able to initiate reflection and discussion, perhaps through clinical supervision, then do so. If support is not available to you then consider setting it up.

There is a clear clinical and moral imperative to deal directly with ethical issues of resuscitation. There is no short-cut to ethical decision-making. It is either arrogant or ignorant to believe that there is. Nurses, in particular, need to feel, through their own ethical understanding and reasoning, that it is right and proper to raise these issues for open discussion. In order to do so you must have insight into your personal beliefs and be properly informed about ethical reasoning. Above all, you must know your patients as individuals and develop trusting and honest relationships in which their preferences and their underlying beliefs and values can be comfortably explored and accommodated. If you have missed the opportunity to do so, the patient is held hostage to clinical indecision and vulnerable to indignity. You may or may not believe that that is a fate worse than death.

REFERENCES

Beauchamp T I, Childress J F 1983 Principles of biomedical ethics. Oxford University Press, Oxford

Bentham J 1968 An introduction to the principles of morals and legislation. In: Warnock M (ed.) Utilitarianism. Fontana Library, Glasgow

BMA 1993 Medical ethics today: its practice and philosophy. BMJ Publishing Group, London

Declaration of Helsinki 1964, revised 1975 Recommendations guiding physicians in biomedical research involving human subjects. Adopted by the 18th World Medical Assembly (WMA) in 1964 and revised by the 29th WMA in Tokyo, 1975

Department of Health 1999 The Health Bill. The Stationery Office, London, Cll 19–25

Gillon R 1992 Philosophical medical ethics. John Wiley, Chichester

Harris J 1985 The values of life. Routledge, London

Kant I 1948 Groundwork of the metaphysic of morals. In: Paton H J (ed.) The moral law. Hutchinson University Library, London

Miles S H 1994 Medical futility. In Monagle J F, Thomasma D C (eds) Health care ethics: critical issues. Aspen Publishers, Maryland, pp 233–240

Mill J S 1962 Utilitarianism. In: Warnock M (ed.) Utilitarianism. William Collins, Oxford

Monagle J F, Thomasma D C 1994 Health care ethics: critical issues. Aspen Publishers, Maryland

Rawls J 1976 A theory of justice. Oxford University Press, Oxford

Resuscitation Council (UK), BMA and RCN 1993 Decisions relating to cardiopulmonary resuscitation. Joint Statement from the Resuscitation Council (UK) BMA and RCN, London

Singleton J, McLaren S 1995 Ethical foundations of health care. Mosby, London

UKCC 1992 Code of professional conduct for the nurse, midwife and health visitor. UKCC, London

UKCC 1996 Guidelines for professional practice. UKCC, London

Williams A 1992 Cost-effectiveness analysis: is it ethical? Journal of Medical Ethics 18: 7–11

Legal aspects of resuscitation

Shiona Gardiner

3

■ CONTENTS

INTRODUCTION

I am not going to discuss what a cardiac arrest is and how it has been used/abused in the last 35 years. Neither am I going to refer to how people (mainly physicians) come to make their decision(s) regarding who should and should not be resuscitated (except for attempting to set it within the legal context). However, I will be referring to the previous chapter on Ethics and attempting to put that into some kind of legal framework.

WHERE DOES THE LAW COME FROM?

The law in the UK comes from three main sources: the common law, Statute law and case law (which is essentially the judges interpreting Statute and common law). Statute law is the passing of Acts of Parliament. These Acts begin as Bills and the Bills emanate either from the government's agenda or from private members of either House. Once the Bills have been debated in the House of Commons, they progress into the House of Lords. The debate moves between these two houses until agreement is reached as to intention and wording. They are then given the official sanction of the Queen to become Acts of Parliament. In the hierarchy of law, Statute is always highest and ought to be followed.

There is no Act of Parliament governing either resuscitation or dying, although various attempts have been made to put euthanasia in the Statute Book. In 1936, the Voluntary Euthanasia (Legalisation) Bill was introduced in the House of Lords by Lord Moynihan and Lord Dawson. This Bill failed to reach the Statute Book. In 1969, another Bill was introduced and it too was unsuccessful. The Incurable Patients Bill, introduced in 1976, suffered a similar fate and in 1990, Roland Boyes introduced a Bill to the House of Commons to permit voluntary euthanasia. The vote for that Bill was 35 for and 101 against, so, as there is no Statute to guide us, we are left with common law and case law governing this thorny issue.

To resuscitate someone means that one actively has to do something. In the UK, it is illegal to do something to someone, if they are competent adult beings, without their consent. Even with their consent it can be illegal – see *R v Brown* (1994), which was a case about homosexuals who were engaged in sadomasochistic acts between consenting adults, and *R v Wilson* (1996), concerning a husband branding a wife with a cigarette end.

If we lay hands on someone without their consent, we could be guilty of the common law offence of battery or of trespass to the person. However, health professionals do it all the time, when taking temperatures, blood pressures, etc. Why are we not called in by the police and criminally charged or sued by the patient?

The answer is that most patients do not know much about what has happened. Depending on the result of whatever it was that was done to them, they are either quite grateful or they do not know that they can complain, although that is not always the case. More and more patients are becoming aware of their rights and they now know what do.

A landmark judgement in the appeal case of *R v Collins and others ex parte S* (1998) was reported in the Independent newspaper. In this case, a pregnant woman was given a Caesarean section in 1996 without her consent, using the Mental Health Act 1983. Without the Caesarean both she and her baby would have probably died. In 1998, with both mother and baby alive and well, the mother appealed the decision and in this appeal it was stated that even where medical intervention appears necessary in order to save someone's life, it was not to be done unless the patient gave consent. If the patient is of sound mind and able to make decisions, however irrational they may appear to the health professional, the patient ought to be left to make them and they should be abided by.

RESUSCITATION?

One naïvely may think that there is not a patient in their right mind who would sue a health professional for 'bringing them back from the dead'. However, this is not so. I can recall many patients who were very bitter about being resuscitated.

In the previous chapter, autonomy was discussed and that is what this is about: the ability to make your own choices, to steer your own course and not to be led, however well-meaning, in some direction that you do not want to go. However, in order to make a choice there must be information and that is the nurse's role – to give the patients information.

In every nursing model, there is a section about death or dying: *use it*. Discuss this with your patients. They will want to contribute to this fundamental part of their life. Death is a very difficult subject to raise, but it is the only inevitable thing in our lives. The only thing we do not know about death is when it will actually happen. Everyone who comes into hospital worries about dying, regardless of the reason for their visit. As nurses, we need to acknowledge that. Tell them all about cardiopulmonary resuscitation (CPR). Ask them if, in the extremely unlikely event of their heart stopping, they would want to be resuscitated. Take your cue from them. Never presume that someone prefers living to dying. Discuss it with them and then record their decision. Share that decision with all other health professionals.

QUESTIONS

Resuscitation raises many questions. I have itemized five of these below and will attempt to answer them.

1. What about the doctor?
2. What about the patient who does not want to know?
3. Would I be deemed negligent if I did not resuscitate someone?
4. Would I be trespassing on someone's body if I resuscitated them and I knew they did not want that to happen?
5. If I cannot ask the patient, can I ask the next of kin?

What about the doctor?

The doctor may have told you that you are not to tell the patient anything about their diagnosis or prognosis. However, do we lie to the patient? Far better to say that it is something you are not entitled to tell, but the doctor has more information (if that is, indeed, the case), and be there with the patient when they ask the doctor, listening to what the doctor has to say. Prompt the patient if need be, to ensure that they understand what the doctor is telling them.

The doctor may say that it is the health professional's choice whether to resuscitate or not. However, it should be the patient's choice, and only the patient's. That is, of course, if they are given the choice or opportunity. What patients do, in essence, if given that choice is make what one could construe as an 'Advanced Directive'. I will elaborate on advanced directives a little later in the chapter.

Health professionals often hide behind the defence of necessity when they do things without the consent of the patient. In the main, the result is a happy, grateful, living patient – one who probably did not want to die. But what about the person who is possibly tired of living? Should they not, at least, have a say in what is going to be done to them without their consent?

The other side of the coin is the patient who may be designated 'do not resuscitate' (DNR). Do they know? I think that they usually do not because this would mean health professionals having to justify their decisions on a patient being too old, too frail, or having a medical condition such that it would be futile to resuscitate. However, is there really anything wrong in this? Everyone knows that choices have to be made regarding who gets what. What is wrong with publishing the criteria? Can the decision-making process be challenged? It could, but provided that the criteria used were not bizarre or out of the ordinary, it probably would not make any difference. You may have heard of, or read about the case of *Bolam* v *Friern Hospital Management Committee* (1957). This case involved the question of negligence and it was said by Justice McNair that:

> 'a doctor is not guilty of negligence if he has acted in accordance with a practice accepted as proper by a responsible body of medical men skilled in that particular art'

Putting it another way, a doctor is not negligent if they are acting in accordance with such a practice, even if there is a body of opinion that takes the contrary view. At the same time, that does not mean that a medical person can obstinately carry on with some technique if it has been proved to be contrary to what is substantially the whole of informed medical opinion.

From the above, one can see that if a patient, or more probably their relatives, challenged the doctor's decision not to resuscitate (if, indeed, they ever found out that they had a DNR order in their notes), the doctor would have a reasonable defence if they could say that the decision was in accordance with a 'responsible body of medical men skilled in that particular art'. This principle has been repeated time and time again in cases since 1957 and it was in *Bolitho* v *City and Hackney Health Authority* (1992) that Lord Justice Dillon took this concept that little bit further by stating:

> 'In my judgement, the court could only adopt the approach of Sachs LJ and reject medical opinion on the ground that the reasons of one group of doctors do not really stand up to analysis, if the court, fully conscious of its own lack of medical knowledge and clinical experience, was none the less clearly satisfied that the views of that group of doctors were *Wednesbury* unreasonable'

i.e. *views such as no reasonable body of doctors could have held* (my italics); see also *Associated Provincial Picture Houses Ltd* v *Wednesbury Corp.* (1947) 2 All ER 680, [1948] 1 KB 223.

What about the patient who does not want to know?

We all know that there are still patients who trust in the health system and do not want to know what is happening to them. The first thing you have to do is ascertain whether that is truly the case. This takes experience and tact; it is not something one learns overnight. They may be saying one thing verbally but their body language may be transmitting something else; gently probe to find out. Once you have probed and come to a decision about the veracity of their statement, *record it*. Try to get the patient to sign in their notes that they agree with what you have written. Record whether they did or did not want to sign in agreement. If the patient truly does not want to know then whatever you do to them must be in accordance with good practice. However, you must always attempt to explain to your patient and not just assume that they have not changed their mind.

Would I be deemed negligent if I did not resuscitate someone?

In order to prove negligence three things must be present:

1. There must be a duty of care.
2. You must breach that duty of care by act or omission i.e. do something that you should not have done or do it incorrectly (act) or not do something that you should have done (omission).
3. Harm must be caused to the patient directly because of your breach.

There is usually a duty of care between a health professional and their patient, but does that duty involve resuscitating them? This is a moot point. Again, with reference to *Bolam* v *Friern Hospital Management Committee* (1957) and *Bolitho* v *City and Hackney Health Authority* (1992), the question is, would another nurse or body of nurses resuscitate this person? If the answer to that question is yes, you should resuscitate and not to do so would be negligent if your action of not resuscitating would cause harm to the patient. One could say that by not resuscitating, you have deprived that patient of their life, but would that patient have died anyway, despite your efforts? Look again at the statistics regarding successful recovery. Can someone claim damages for a loss of chance? Lord Mackay of Clashfern in the case of *Hotson* v *East Berkshire Area Health Authority* (1987) considered it 'unwise in the present case to lay it down as a rule that a plaintiff could never succeed by proving loss of a chance in a medical negligence case'. Moreover, Lord Diplock in *Mallett* v *McMonagle* (1970) stated that

'In determining what did happen in the past a court decides on the balance of probabilities. Anything that is more probable than not it treats as certain.'

It appears from the above that a patient, through his relatives, could indeed, claim for loss of chance if it can be proved that, on a balance of probabilities, the patient would have survived had resuscitative measures been taken.

Would I be trespassing on someone's body if I resuscitated them and I knew they did not want that to happen?

Theoretically the answer to this is yes, bearing in mind the concept of autonomy and consent and taking into account the recent appeal case of *R* v *Collins and others ex parte S* (1998). Nevertheless, what would actually happen? Most patients, as mentioned above, are very pleased to find themselves alive, if a little sore. However, if you extrapolate the decision in *R* v *Collins and others ex parte S* (1998) to include resuscitation, it appears that they can sue you for saving their lives if they did not give you their consent. The case mentioned was about a surgical procedure that required consent and the consent had been deliberately withheld. Resuscitation, one could argue, is an entirely different situation, since cardiac arrest happens spontaneously and is life threatening without intervention. In *R* v *Collins and others ex parte S* (1998) Lord Justice Judge stated that there would be occasions when an individual lacked the capacity to make decisions about whether or not to consent to treatment and on these occasions the medical practitioners had to act in the patient's best interests. This makes it even more important to find out beforehand what it is the patient actually wants to happen.

If I cannot ask the patient, can I ask the next of kin?

Consider who has to give consent for anything else – the patient. Relatives are a wonderful source of information when we need to know about certain things in order to care for our patients, but it is a well-known fact that even very close couples know less than they think they know about each other. The best person to ask is always the patient if possible. Always remember that the next of kin may have an interest in whether a patient lives or dies. In law, relatives have no right to give or withhold consent.

This brings us to the status of Advanced Directives or 'Living Wills'. It would appear that if a person wrote their wishes down and had it witnessed by two people, and had discussed it with their GP, then it could be valid. The British Medical Association has published guidelines for the writing of an Advanced Directive as has the Voluntary Euthanasia Society. The problem with Advanced Directives is that they have never been tested in court. Until then, one cannot state that they are legally binding documents. On balance, however, if there is such a document, *follow it.*

CONCLUSION

In summary I suggest that you always attempt to find out what your patients want to happen to them, however difficult that may be. All patients are unique human beings and the art is to communicate with them in order to assess their needs and wishes for the future. Find out what they want to happen. Discuss with them the feasibility of that happening. It is their life and their death – let them decide.

CASES CITED

Associated Provincial Picture Houses Ltd v *Wednesbury Corp.* 1947 2 All ER 680, 1948 1 KB 223
Bolam v *Friern Hospital Management Committee* 1957 1 BMLR 1
Bolitho v *City and Hackney Health Authority* 1992 13 BMLR 111
Hotson v *East Berkshire Area Health Authority* 1987 3WLR 232
Mallett v *McMonagle* 1970 AC 166
R v *Brown* 1994 1 AC 212
R v *Collins and others ex parte S* 1998 Reported in the Independent 12th May 1998
R v *Wilson* 1996 2 Cr. App. R. 241

The role of the nurse in resuscitation attempts in hospitals

4

Annie Chellel

■ CONTENTS

INTRODUCTION

Resuscitation is taught in artificially simulated situations that are controlled and manipulated to enable those attending to rehearse their skills and increase their knowledge. Resuscitation in reality is far more dramatic in its urgency, demanding in its complexity and difficult because of the distress it causes. The shock experienced on first seeing a resuscitation attempt will be vividly remembered, for it is a violent and technologically dominated intervention at the moment of death. For nurses this constitutes the antithesis of the peaceful, dignified and pain-free death that we would wish for our patients, our loved ones and indeed ourselves. Few of those who are resuscitated survive to be discharged home from hospital (see chapter 8); however 'do not resuscitate orders' remain the exception in acute hospitals, despite claims that there are identifiable groups for whom resuscitation is a nugatory and costly exercise (Murphy & Finucane 1993). How then are nurses to reconcile themselves to this brutal procedure in which patients are denied a peaceful death on the strength of little evidence of its efficacy? My personal belief is that nurses understand the importance of hope in caring for a dying patient and express this throughout resuscitation attempts by maintaining respect for the dignity of the patient, compassion for the relatives and support for other patients. This enables nurses to maintain their perspective and cope with the death of patients (Page & Meerabeau 1996).

The purpose of this chapter is to explore the role of the nurse in resuscitation attempts in hospital. I begin by describing the complexity of the role of the nurse, which is created by multiple and often conflicting demands on nursing time and attention. I then show that this is the inevitable consequence of the unique nursing perspective in which physical care and scientific knowledge are combined with compassion and caring. The sudden collapse of a patient creates an urgent demand for rapid clinical decision-making, based on sound professional judgement and carefully considered priorities. The urgent need to save a life requires the highest quality nursing, if the needs of the collapsed patient, medical and nursing colleagues, the relatives and the other patients, are to be met. This chapter is divided into two sections: the first describes the diversity of roles taken by the nurse in resuscitation attempts and the second explores some of the theoretical concepts of nursing which inform that role. This will be achieved through examining the foundations of the professional judgements made during arrest situations, in order to illuminate the complexity, the subtlety and the humanist perspective of the nursing role in resuscitation.

THE DIVERSITY OF NURSES' ROLES DURING RESUSCITATION ATTEMPTS

I have argued for some time that the responsibilities of nurses in resuscitation attempts are more complex and more demanding than those of doctors (Chellel 1993). Doctors, who run in to treat collapsed patients, usually find equipment ready to hand and nursing staff who will support and assist them as appropriate. The medical role is to strive to revive the patient using their knowledge and experience of guidelines based, for the most part at least, on scientific research. In the event of success, the doctor must transfer and follow the patient to intensive care and in the event of failure, they must know when to stop, speak briefly to the family and return to their other medical responsibilities. This division of labour is, of course, entirely appropriate, since medicine is concerned primarily with the pathophysiology of cardiorespiratory arrest, its diagnosis and its treatment in order to save life. Nursing, however, while sharing the scientific approach to the physical treatment of arrested patients, is also concerned with the effects of the pathophysiology and its treatment not only on an individual, but also on those around them. Whatever the outcome, nurses must deal with the resuscitation attempt itself and its consequences before, during and after the arrival of the advanced life support (ALS) team. The focus of nursing in resuscitation attempts is therefore also concerned with the care of a dying patient, whose needs are psychological and spiritual. The human consequences of sudden death will affect all who are involved either personally or professionally. This caring aspect of the nurse's role has the inevitable consequence of making resuscitation a rather more prolonged and more complex event for nurses, who have other, simultaneous, responsibilities in differing and sometimes conflicting areas. These are shown diagrammatically in Figure 4.1, and are discussed in greater detail below.

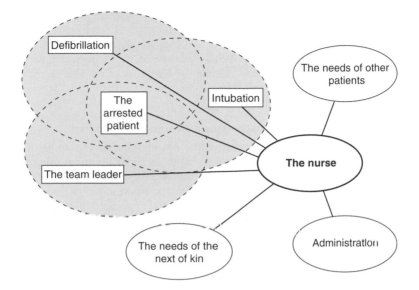

Fig. 4.1 The diversity of roles and responsibilities for nurses during resuscitation attempts.

Responsibilities to the arrested patient

From the outset, nurses must respond at once to the physical needs of the arrested patient by diagnosing the arrest, summoning the help of the ALS team and instigating basic life support (BLS). They must then gather all the necessary ward equipment and take it to the bedside, and clear the area ready for the team to manoeuvre. In my experience, ward equipment (suction, oxygen, drugs and defibrillator) is not always 'state of the art', ergonomically designed, all-in-one, sleek, efficient, minimalist or light. Often, it consists of several separate bits and pieces, such as an oxygen cylinder or suction apparatus that, although labelled portable, may be large, old, heavy and unwieldy. Nurses are responsible for maintaining whatever life-saving equipment is kept on the ward in a state of readiness. They should know what equipment they have, where it is kept and how to use it in an emergency. Nurses are accountable to their patients according to the Code of Professional Conduct and have a duty to ensure that no act or omission on their part is detrimental to the patient (UKCC 1992a, clause 2). All nurses should ensure that they are able to resuscitate should the need arise, and they must therefore be skilled and knowledgeable in resuscitation techniques. Nurses, like any other health care professional, may be called upon to resuscitate patients, friends or family, at work, at home or at social occasions. Resuscitation training programmes are now widely available in most hospitals since resuscitation training officer posts have become more widespread. The Resuscitation Council (UK) provides certification for both trainers and courses, to ensure uniformity of course content and to maintain the standard of teaching. During resuscitation attempts, the priority of nursing care is the physical needs of the patient, and nurses should know the algorithms of BLS and ALS (see chapters 6 and 7). Nurses, at the same time, may be caring for a dying patient and this aspect of their care will be discussed later in this chapter in the section on the theoretical aspects underlying nursing care in resuscitation.

Responsibilities to the advanced life support team

On the arrival of the team, nurses must assist and support them as necessary; by preparing drugs, assisting with intubation, defibrillation, maintaining cardiac compressions and ventilation and keeping a record of events. At later stages, they may assist with sending of blood samples for analysis and organizing a transfer to an intensive care unit, or dealing with the death of one of their patients. Inexperienced nurses need both teaching and support during and after the event to enable them to develop their skills and knowledge regarding resuscitation. They may also need encouragement to discuss the incident and reflect upon the emotional stress of dealing with the death of a patient.

The old professional boundaries are breaking down. Substitution is becoming more widespread in an effort to achieve greater cost efficiency (Richardson and Maynard 1995, p. 17). *The Scope of Professional Practice* (UKCC 1992b) allows nurses to carry out any procedure for the benefit of the patient, if they have received the necessary education and training. Since more nurses are fully trained in ALS, they may now undertake any of the team roles in resuscitation, such as peripheral venous cannulation, defibrillation or team leadership, which were once taken only by doctors.

Nurses have a duty to collaborate with doctors and other hospital staff, such as operating department assistants, to work as a team according to local protocol and immediate need, to ensure that everything possible is done quickly and efficiently, to save a life (see chapters 6 and 7). It should be remembered that the algorithms are guidelines and may need to be adapted to meet the requirements of an individual resuscitation attempt. Each is unique because of not only the age and history of the patient, and the pathologies leading to the arrest, but also the time, location and context of the arrest. Nurses must be intelligent in their understanding of the algorithms in order to be able to adapt them to each situation and work under pressure with people they may not know. However, nurses should remember that their major contribution in resuscitation attempts is their knowledge of the patient, gained from thorough nursing assessment as part of the nursing process. It is this knowledge that allows nurses to contribute to decision-making by giving a brief but essential history of the arrest to the team leader and also by providing background knowledge of the patient's wishes, their overall condition, progress and prognosis. This will be discussed in detail in the second section of this chapter.

Responsibilities to other patients

Nurses still have responsibilities to other patients who are inevitably distressed by the drama being acted out in front of them. Curtains do not act as a barrier to sound and nearby patients are often only too aware of what is going on. These patients may be witness to a fight against death, in which they too may be personally engaged, since their own pathology has brought them into hospital: this terrible event forces them to face the possibility that it might also happen to them. They may have struck up an acquaintance with the arrested patient, or may even have witnessed the arrest and summoned the first nurse on the scene. All those involved with resuscitation events are inevitably reminded of their own mortality, for this drama is like a stone cast into the water, whose ripples spread to touch many lives. Nurses must explain simply and truthfully what is going on and try to comfort nearby patients and reassure them that everything possible is being done to save a life. Ward nurses need first to recognize that nearby patients suffer fear, distress and anxiety, and second to accept that all patients and more inexperienced staff may be profoundly affected by resuscitation attempts and require some support.

The ward work does not cease while resuscitation attempts are being made and other patients' needs must still be met. Indeed, there may be other seriously ill patients on the ward whose observation and treatment require a high nurse dependency. This may create a conflict of need for the nurses. The safety of other patients must be ensured and the essential work of the shift maintained during the arrest. Nurses must make carefully considered professional judgements to prioritize and restructure the shift work at a time when they are under pressure, both physically and emotionally. The arrest will have taken up a considerable amount of nursing time, often requiring the complete attention of two nurses. After the event, nurses must clear away the inevitable mess and ensure that the resuscitation equipment and drugs are replaced immediately in case they are needed again. We have all heard tales of two arrests occurring at once, and this is no myth – many of us have experienced it.

The Patient's next of Kin

Nurses are often required to contact the next of kin, if they are not already present, and call them to the hospital. This should be done as soon as possible after the arrest call has been made to allow the relatives a chance to see their loved one before they die or are transferred to intensive care. Speaking to families or significant others under this circumstance, requires sensitivity. It is essential to tell the truth clearly and simply and to be aware of how shocking and distressing it is to be telephoned with such dreadful news (Wright 1996, p. 14; see also chapter 5). It is a simple, but sound rule that nurses should treat relatives as they themselves would wish to be treated, were their own mother, father, brother or child to suffer a cardiorespiratory arrest. These shocked, frightened and anxious people will remember this occasion for the rest of their lives and we have a duty to try to help them through this terrible event so that healing can take place and their lives be restored.

Conflict may arise for the nurse when the patient's family arrives. They will be very upset and will clearly need a nurse to meet them, sit with them and explain what is happening. They also need privacy (Wright 1996, p. 16) to help them cope with their distress. However, the immediate demands of the resuscitation attempt itself will take priority and nurses may have to leave them waiting outside the ward. Relatives may wish to be present at the resuscitation attempt. Nurses should be aware that if they do wish to be present, all staff must be aware of the implications for the patient, the resuscitating team and the relative involved. These issues are discussed fully in chapter 5. The question of who is the next of kin and whether they are indeed the most important person to the arrested patient may also create a conflict for the nurse. Nurses must establish when admitting and assessing their patients, who they would like to be called in the event of an emergency. There is little worse than having a patient arrest and discovering that the admitting nurse has failed to record the name and telephone number of the person the patient wanted to be informed. Nurses should ensure, as part of the assessment process, that the wishes of both the patient and their next of kin are sought and that this important information is recorded in the nursing notes. For further discussion on the care of relatives please refer to chapter 5.

Ward Administration

Nursing records must be written as soon as possible after the event (as required by law). A full account of the arrest and its treatment, including the names of personnel who responded and the time critical events took place should be recorded in the patient's nursing record. This record should include the time that next of kin were informed and the point at which they were able to see the patient. Nurses may also be involved in the collection of data for audit or research purposes according to local requirements, ideally following the Utstein template (see chapter 8). In the meantime, other ward work does not disappear, and all other administrative duties must be taken up again. It is not easy, immediately after a resuscitation attempt, to deal with phone calls, hospital staff and patient enquiries from people who do not know what has just happened. The rest of the hospital continues its endless round of activity, oblivious of the drama that has just taken place. Bed management, the off-duty, writing up of care plans and all the other details of ward administration, must be picked up again where they were left off. However, for nurses and for other patients, it can seem disrespectful and insensitive to carry on as if nothing had happened with no time for an intervening period of recovery and mourning for the passing of a life.

THE THEORETICAL FOUNDATIONS OF NURSING PROFESSIONAL JUDGEMENT IN CARDIOPULMONARY RESUSCITATION ATTEMPTS

Nurses, when dealing with resuscitation attempts in hospitals, are subject to a most rigorous and public test of their nursing skills. They are required to make many clinical decisions rapidly in order to meet the diverse demands made upon them described in the first section of this chapter (see Fig. 4.1). This requires sound professional judgement, which is the product of the invisible cognitive process of clinical decision-making. In this process, the nurse's personal knowledge, beliefs, values and experience are brought together, interpreted and applied to the clinical context. This context includes the factors illustrated in Figure 4.1, as well as the arrested patient and the other professionals involved in the resuscitation attempt (Fig. 4.2).

The interpretative process, which combines the underlying components of nursing professional judgement, is rapid, fluent and almost subconscious. The underpinning aspects of professional judgement illustrated in Figure 4.2 constitute the theoretical domain of nursing. This creates the humanist perspective that lies at the heart of nursing practice. The elements of epistemology, philosophy, ethics and experience may be both eclectic and diverse, but their disparity is no obstacle to their combination. Indeed,

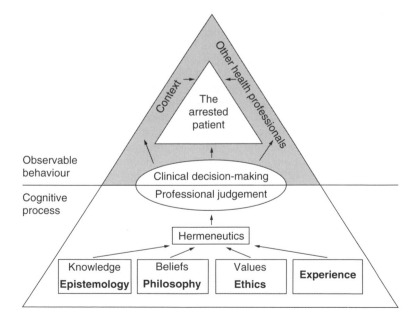

Fig. 4.2 Theoretical aspects of nursing and their relationship to professional judgement in resuscitation attempts. Adapted from Endacott & Chellel (1996), with permission.

nursing practice is the expression of their influence, for they become so closely interwoven that they overlap and merge to create a fluid whole when making professional nursing judgements. This fusion is difficult to portray and so, for the sake of expedience, I will attempt to deal with each separately, although the separation is a literary convenience rather than a reflection of the reality of clinical decision-making.

Epistemology

The epistemology or knowledge base of nursing is eclectic, and has been described as a combination of art and science (Carper 1978, Rose & Parker 1994). Scientific knowledge is that which is empirically derived and, for nurses, as in resuscitation, it is often borrowed from the more positivist disciplines of medicine and its related fields of physiology and pharmacology. Nurses must know and understand the pharmacological treatment of cardiac arrest (see chapter 7) and the electrophysiological rationales for defibrillation (see chapter 10). They should also be aware of the scientific basis of the algorithms (see chapters 6 and 7) in order to be able to apply them intelligently. Nurses should also be prepared to contribute to the development of this scientific knowledge by carrying out nursing research, collecting audit data as required (see chapter 8), or contributing to collaborative research whenever possible. It is, of course, incumbent upon nurses to maintain and improve their knowledge and skills as required by the UKCC (1992a, clause 3).

The 'artistic' knowledge of nursing, however, is that which differentiates our discipline from others and is concerned with imagination, intuition and creativity (Appleton 1993, Chinn & Kramer 1995, p. 10). It is knowledge of the person and knowledge of nursing, combined with the application of scientific nursing knowledge, which enables nursing to make its unique contribution to patient care, described by Marks-Maran (1997, p. 108) as nursing wisdom. Nursing knowledge of the patient is acquired through proximity, the creation of a therapeutic nurse–patient relationship and through continuous nursing assessment (Radwin 1996). The therapeutic relationship is based upon mutual trust, commitment and caring (Morse 1991). It is the basis of our role as patient advocate and, as such, is perhaps our most valuable contribution to the multidisciplinary team in resuscitation attempts. Nurses should give the brief history of the patient's condition and collapse and inform the team leader of any other relevant information concerning the patient's wishes, beliefs or expectations. These personal details give the team leader a fuller picture of the patient as an individual, rather than as a cardiac arrest case, and enable them to make more informed and appropriate decisions.

The nurse draws upon a complex synthesis of knowledge from both the art and science of nursing to inform the rapid clinical decisions made in arrest situations. The nursing contribution requires practice skills and advanced knowledge of resuscitation, its causes and its treatment as well as individual knowledge of the patient as a person, their condition, their understanding, their situation, their expectations and their wishes.

Philosophy

Philosophy is what we believe about the nature of life and death. The philosophy of nursing which lies at the heart of any nursing context may have been explored and articulated by nurses in a ward philosophy. Alternatively, a nursing model may be used which is based on a theorist's philosophical perception of the metaparadigms of person, health, environment and nursing (Chinn & Kramer 1995, p. 40). Perhaps the most widely used model in this country is the Roper–Logan–Tierney model (Fraser 1996, p. 13). One of the five elements of this model is the 12 activities of living, which include 'Fear of Dying', as an area for nursing assessment and intervention (Roper et al. 1996, p. 395). Nurses should be familiar with the philosophy of the model they use and consider its relationship to their ward philosophy, as well as to their own beliefs about the nature and purpose of nursing within their clinical context. In resuscitation, these philosophical issues are particularly important because a dying patient is being nursed: in this situation, spiritual care becomes a priority which must compete with the other demands on nursing time and attention (Fig. 4.1). It is our philosophy of nursing that shapes priorities and clinical decisions when caring for patients being resuscitated.

Spiritual care

Nurses should be aware of the culture of their patients and the religious beliefs and practices that form part of that culture. In our cosmopolitan society, nurses may now encounter patients of any of the world's religions. The patient's spiritual beliefs are particularly relevant as death approaches and the nurse should be aware of any religious requirements which may affect the nursing care of the patient before and after death. The specific treatment of the body may vary considerably for each religion and nurses must be sensitive to the ritual practices of the patient's faith in order to meet the spiritual needs of both the patient and their family. Many hospitals provide this information in leaflets; alternatively, nurses can refer to the *Marsden Manual* (Mallett and Bailey 1996) which offers guidelines for these requirements.

Those who have a religion draw comfort from their faith (Neuberger 1987, p. 2), and the presence of ritual under a theological guide of their faith, can help the patient and their distressed relatives to face death. Their spiritual needs should be met if at all practicable, although this is difficult in the emergency of a resuscitation attempt. Thorough nursing assessment should include enquiry into the spiritual beliefs and needs of the patient: they should be discussed and recorded on admission, or later when the nurse and patient have established a trusting relationship.

There are difficulties in discussing death and resuscitation with patients who are terminally ill or dying within the context of the acute setting. However, I would suggest these difficulties relate to the nurse's anxieties about discussing death rather than the patient's. The patient's wishes must be discovered and respected in order for nurses to demonstrate real respect for patient dignity and autonomy. It is only by discussing the patient's wishes in the event of their sudden collapse that nurses can take the role of patient advocate either during resuscitation attempts, or when instigating or reversing 'do not resuscitate orders'. In the case of emergency admission or admission of unconscious patients, this is not possible. However, the presence of a spiritual guide as death approaches can be helpful, even if from a different faith, and in my experience hospital chaplains can offer a great deal of solace to patients and relatives at this time. They can also be a great support to nurses who are faced with the conflicting demands of spiritual care for the patient and their distressed relatives, and the more immediate physical demands of the resuscitation attempt itself.

Surviving patients and the near-death experience

I have nursed perhaps eight to ten patients over the last 20 years, who described to me their recollections of what they experienced while being resuscitated.

The patients mentioned in case histories 4.1 and 4.2 were describing what are now called near-death experiences (NDEs), which have been the subject of scientific research for many years. There are two main interpretations of these accounts; the first postulates that they are the result of cerebral hypoxia in a dying brain, while the second suggests that they are paranormal experiences providing evidence of life after death (Blackmore 1993, pp. 3–4). Sabom (1982) analysed data from 116 interviews in his study of patients who had survived a near-death event. NDEs were reported by 40% of these patients and Sabom categorizes them into three types. The first is

---

Case history 4.1

Bill asked me, 'Do you believe in ghosts Sister?' He was sitting in a chair awaiting transfer to the ward after a lengthy weaning process from ventilation in intensive care, following a cardiac arrest in the accident and emergency department. I replied that having never seen one I couldn't be sure either way, but did not rule out the possibility of their existence. I wondered why he had asked that question. Bill then said that while being resuscitated he had been separated from his body, which he had seen lying on the trolley surrounded by doctors, nurses and equipment and had begun willingly to move towards a bright, peaceful and welcoming light. He saw his uncle, who had had been like a father to him. Bill was unafraid and felt great joy at seeing his uncle who had died some 5 years previously. Bill's uncle spoke to him and explained that it was not yet his time and that he should return. He took Bill by the hand and led him back to his body. I sat and talked to Bill for some time about his experience and explained that his was not the first account I had heard of what is now called a near-death experience. This seemed to reassure him because the memory of his experience was preying on his mind and he needed to understand what it meant. He was convinced that it was evidence of life after death and this reassured him. He said that he was no longer afraid of dying.

Case history 4.2

Mary was suffering from recurrent ventricular fibrillation following a myocardial infarction. She had been resuscitated many times and said one day after another successful resuscitation that she had something to tell me. She recounted her experience of moving through a dark tunnel towards a bright light which welcomed her and which she wanted to enter. She sensed rather than saw that in the light was a beautiful, peaceful garden. Mary described a feeling that she had a choice to go or to come back. She had chosen to return because she had 'things to do'. Mary said that next time she would not come back. She then called in her family and made her farewells. She also called for some papers from home and made financial arrangements. Mary did arrest again a few days later and we were unable to resuscitate her.

---

the autoscopic, in which the patient leaves the body and sees themself and what is happening to them from above. In this out-of-body state the patient may encounter others known to be dead, or a god-like being with whom they are able to communicate before returning to their bodies. The second is the transcendental type in which the patient experiences an 'out of this world place' through which they move from darkness to light or some place of great beauty. Some experience a life review and again encounters with others are reported and finally a return to the body. The third is a combined NDE in which elements of both autoscopic and transcendental NDEs are experienced. These experiences were highly significant events for the patients who had them and they have the effect of lessening fear of death and creating a more positive attitude to life.

In a study by Greyson (1993), NDEs were reported by 76% of 246 individuals who had come close to death. A taxonomy of these experiences was also offered: cognitive elements, which include time distortion, panoramic life review, a sense of sudden understanding and acceleration of thought processes; affective elements, which include feelings of overwhelming peace, well-being, joy and cosmic unity; paranormal elements, which include out of body experiences; and, finally, transcendental elements, which include travel to an unearthly realm and encounters with mystical or deceased figures. Interestingly, Greyson (1993) cites the example of Livingstone's account, written in 1872, while being attacked by a lion in Africa, and Jung's description of an NDE while suffering a heart attack in 1944. Greyson's (1993) research suggests that cardiac arrest appears to be highly correlated with NDEs and their paranormal, affective and transcendental elements. Kellehear (1993) and Morse (1994) suggest that the type of NDE experienced may be culturally determined and there is evidence that for a small number of people they are not pleasant (Greyson & Evans Bush 1992).

Nurses should be aware that NDEs are not uncommon and patients recovering after successful resuscitation may need to discuss them. I always find a quiet moment to ask patients who have been resuscitated if they remember anything about what happened to them. This gives them the opportunity to discuss their NDE, if they have had one. Even those who have not had such an experience are aware that they came very close to dying and will need to come to terms with it. They may need to explore its meaning and make sense of what happened. Vintner (1994) recommends that nurses use their knowledge of the research on NDEs to reassure patients that they are real phenomena and the subject of research. Cole (1993) suggests that nurses should inform patients about NDEs and cites Corocan's (1988) proposal that nurses also need to explore their own attitudes and not seek to explain away patients' accounts. This view is shared by Bucher *et al.* (1997), whose research indicates that nurses are aware of and interested in NDEs but lack specific nursing interventions to help their patients. They suggest that touching the patient being resuscitated and giving them reassurance are both important. These authors also recommend that during the recovery period, the nurse should create a trusting relationship, begin a systematic reorientation to reality and encourage the patient to discuss their recollections of the event. Whatever your beliefs about NDEs, they should be taken seriously. As Blackmore (1996) suggests, it is a matter of personal belief whether you see them as a glimpse of an afterlife or the product of a dying brain, but patients deserve to know what we have learned from research.

Patients who survive resuscitation attempts need to recover spiritually and this is independent of any theological belief. Nurses can help this process by listening to, accepting and respecting the patient's interpretation of the events surrounding the resuscitation attempt. We should not be afraid to discuss philosophical matters with our patients, or their relatives, for death in all its guises is no stranger to nurses who deal with its reality and its consequences as part of their daily practice. There are spiritual and philosophical aspects of the nursing care of dying patients which require recognition if we are to meet our ideal of providing holistic care for those dying patients whose need for such care is the greatest. These aspects, from both the nurse's and the dying patient's perspective, must be taken into account when dealing with patients who are dying or who have survived cardiopulmonary resuscitation.

Ethics

Ethics constitute that branch of philosophy concerned with making judgements about what is good or desirable. The difficulty lies in the fact that such value judgements are highly subjective. Definitions of goodness or 'rightness' are not absolute, but evanescent: they vary according to culture, time, individual opinion, philosophy and the relative congruence between the needs of the individual and those of society. The application of moral principles to individual cases, is therefore fraught with difficulties and contradictions, especially in the case of resuscitation. Nurses should know their patients through the assessment process and the therapeutic nurse–patient relationship: it is this intimate knowledge of the patient that allows the nurse to contribute to ethical decision-making in 'do not resuscitate orders' or at the termination of resuscitation attempts. These issues are discussed fully in chapter 2. My purpose here is to discuss the less controversial but no less complicated ethic of caring. I think I may safely say, without contradiction from most nurses, that caring is a fundamental ideal which lies at the heart of nursing. It has been a subject of scrutiny for many nursing theorists over the last decade. Watson offers a definition of caring as:

'the heart of nursing and the ethical and philosophical foundation of our acts.' (Watson 1994, p. 3)

This author described 10 'carative' factors, including a humanistic altruistic system of values, the instilling of hope, sensitivity to self and others, helping trusting human care relationships (Watson 1988, p. 75). She articulates a claim for caring to be included in nursing's metaparadigm and suggests that it is the foundational ontological substance of nursing which underpins nursing epistemology (Watson 1990).

Roach (1984) described the 'Five Cs' of caring – compassion, competence, confidence, conscience and commitment – and suggested that caring is an ethical imperative of professional nursing. Benner and Wrubel (1989, p. 5) share Watson's view that a caring relationship is central to most nursing interventions.

Eriksson (1992) analysed the structure of caring which is the nurse–patient relationship, the category of caring which is suffering, the motive of caring (the caritas motive) which is human love and the caring communion which is the mutual giving and receiving of care. Whereas Morse *et al.* (1991) carried out a comparative analysis of theories of caring and suggested that five categories emerge: caring as a human trait, caring as moral imperative, caring as an affect, caring as an interpersonal interaction and caring as a therapeutic intervention.

What kind of caring is needed by patients who are being resuscitated and how can that caring be expressed? It has been my experience, when resuscitating, that the patient is assumed to be unconscious and because of the life-threatening urgency of the situation, only the physical treatment of the patient matters. However, research has demonstrated that patients can and do have NDEs and are able to recall what was said during the resuscitation attempts. Although this is usually a reassuring experience, it can also be disturbing. We are also aware that hearing is the last sense to function as consciousness is lost and that resuscitation is a noisy and sometimes chaotic event. It seems that the patient needs reassurance and this can be offered in the form of hope. The nurse assisting with intubation can speak in the patient's ear and address the patient by name, simply explain that they have collapsed, that the medical team is present, and that everything possible is being done to help them. This simple human contact may be the last the patient has. The nurse might also tell them if their family has been called, or are present, and keep them informed at intervals about their treatment. In this way, the nurse can continue to communicate with the unconscious patient as a mark of respect and concern for their predicament. Touching the patient gently by taking the hand or stroking the face or forehead can also convey caring, concern and recognition of the person inside the body being treated. The nurse must be sensitive to the fact that this patient is very close to death and if the attempt is abandoned, the family should be brought in as soon as possible and the equipment removed from their sight. In this way, relatives or loved ones can be with the patient as they die. If this is not possible, a nurse should sit with the patient and hold their hand, for it is my belief that entering and leaving this life should not be accomplished alone. Caring can also be demonstrated when handling the body, by respect for the patient's dignity. I am one of the many nurses who talk to patients as they are being laid out as a gesture of respect and to make this sad task a little easier. Caring should be extended to the family and the patient should look clean and cared for. Equipment should be removed from the bed area before the family approach to say goodbye. Clean linen and a nightgown or pyjama top help to give a more peaceful impression and show consideration for the feelings of the family and the dignity of the patient. I have always found this time immensely sad and have often shed a tear with the family. I do not think this inappropriate: it simply means that although my involvement was professional rather than personal, in some way I share their sense of loss. Nurses do care about their patients, and we should be proud that we do. We need to recognize our involvement in the lives and deaths of our patients. We must continue to explore the nature of professional caring in order to develop ways of being which give it expression, not only for patients, but also for ourselves as human beings and for the profession of nursing.

'The more we understand about caring, the better we shall be able to promote this ordinary yet ennobling and creative art.' (Brykczynska 1997, p. viii)

Experience

Experience has been defined as

' . . . the exposure of people to situations and the development of their skills and knowledge as a result of this exposure.' (Watson 1991)

Watson described four different uses of the word experience to mean exposure to an event, time spent in practice for learning, knowledge gained over a period of time or an event, situation or emotion. Experience of resuscitation incorporates all of those meanings. Nursing experience teaches us the value and fragility of human life; it becomes a part of our nursing knowledge as death gradually becomes familiar to us in all its forms. From each death we learn more about the human condition, from the depths of fear and the horror of pain to the inspiring heights of courage, love and altruism. It is my belief that we are privileged to receive this insight through our intimacy with patients and their families at the moment of death and that it changes us and colours our own beliefs. The experience of caring for dying patients and dealing with death allows nurses to understand better the suffering of their patients and to create meaning within their own lives and personal philosophies (Maeve 1998). This wisdom transforms future practice because the human significance and meaning of clinical situations is more readily interpreted on the basis of that previous experience

Experience of cardiopulmonary resuscitation also gives nurses the opportunity to test and develop their theoretical knowledge, skills and beliefs in practice and, in turn, that experience of practice informs and transforms its underlying cognitive elements. Benner (1984, p. 32) describes the development of expertise through experience, resulting in a fluidity and assurance in practice, which is no longer governed by rules, but by a rapid grasp of meaning and relevance. Schön (1991, p. 42) suggests that it is through reflection that we are able to connect the hard high ground of theory with the swampy lowland of practice. This is particularly pertinent to resuscitation, which is taught in artificial simulations. These lack the drama, complexity, urgency and distress of reality and are therefore limited in their ability to prepare participants for the confusion and occasional chaos of real resuscitation attempts. Each resuscitation attempt is unique and fails to conform to the relative simplicity of simulated teaching events. However, simulated resuscitations offer an essential rehearsal of skills and knowledge within the safety of the classroom, in preparation for the reality. Experience is essential, initially as an observer and then as a participant, in each of the diverse nursing roles in resuscitation, until the experienced nurse is able to use that experience in making sound and compassionate clinical decisions.

CONCLUSION

I have tried, in this chapter to illuminate the diverse and demanding roles of the nurse involved in resuscitation attempts. This is the inevitable result of the nursing perspective, which regards these events not only as cardiopulmonary arrest and its urgent physical treatment, but also as a dramatic and intensely human event with emotional, spiritual and philosophical significance for all those involved. The nursing perspective is unique in its application to all of these elements as legitimate areas of nursing responsibility. The following key points have been made:

1. The role of the nurse in resuscitation attempts in hospitals is extremely complex and diverse. The multiple demands on nursing time are often simultaneous and occasionally conflicting: the nurse must meet the needs of the arrested patient, the attending medical staff, the family of the arrested patient and other patients. Inexperienced nursing and medical staff need both teaching and support.

2. Sophisticated clinical decision-making is required to prioritize and meet these demands. This requires sound professional judgement, in which individual interpretation of nursing epistemology, philosophy and experience is applied to the unique clinical context of a resuscitation attempt.

3. Patients who suffer a cardiorespiratory arrest require urgent physical treatment of the cardiorespiratory arrest and spiritual care. This requires sound scientific knowledge, effective teamwork and compassionate and

sensitive nursing. Caring and the recognition of spirituality are central concepts to nursing the dying, before, during and after the resuscitation attempt.

4. This nursing care is based upon knowledge of the patient acquired through thorough assessment and the creation of a therapeutic nurse–patient relationship. This enables the nurse to demonstrate caring and respect for the patient, to act as their advocate and to deal with the human consequences of resuscitation.

5. The combination of these four elements constitutes the unique contribution of the nurse in cardiopulmonary resuscitation.

We witness many forms of death in our nursing careers but the most violent occurs in resuscitation. We cannot know the hour, the place, or the manner of our demise, nor can we know what we will feel at that time. We can only be certain that the moment must surely come to us all when death is both imminent and inevitable. The illumination we seek into that final human experience does not emerge from the quantitative research of doctors nor yet from the qualitative research of nurses, but from the inspired and imaginative work of a poet.

> 'This is my play's last scene, here heavens appoint
> My pilgrimage's last mile; and my race
> Idly yet swiftly run, hath this last pace,
> My span's last inch, my minute's latest point
> And gluttonous death, will instantly unjoint
> My body and soul, and I shall sleep a space,
> But my ever waking part shall see that face
> Whose fear already shakes my every joint'
> John Donne (1572–1631) *Divine Meditations* No. 6

REFERENCES

Appleton C 1993 The art of nursing: the experience of patients and nurses. Journal of Advanced Nursing 18:892–899
Benner P 1984 From novice to expert. Addison Wesley, London
Benner P, Wrubel J 1989 The primacy of caring. Addison Wesley, Wokingham
Blackmore S 1993 Dying to live. Prometheus Books, Amhurst, NY
Blackmore S 1996 Near-death experiences. Journal of the Royal Society of Medicine 89:73–76
Brykczynska G 1997 Caring: the compassion and wisdom of nursing. Arnold, Sevenoaks
Bucher L, Wimbush F, Hardie T, Hayes E 1997 Near death experiences: critical care nurses' attitudes and interventions. Dimensions of Critical Care Nursing 6(4):194–201
Carper B 1978 Fundamental patterns of knowing and nursing. Advances in Nursing Science 1(1):13–23
Chellel A 1993 CPR: the problems and solutions. Nursing Standard 10(7): 33–36
Chinn P, Kramer M 1995 Theory and nursing: a systematic approach, ch 1, 4th edn. Mosby, London
Cole E 1993 The near death experience. Intensive and Critical Care Nursing 9:157–161

Corocan D 1988 Helping patients who have had near death experiences. Nursing 18(11): 34–39. Cited in Cole 1993

Endacott R, Chellel A 1996 Nursing dependency scoring: measuring the total workload. Nursing Standard 10:39–42

Eriksson K 1992 Nursing: the caring practice 'being there', Chapter 13. In: Gaut D (ed.) The presence of caring in nursing. National League for Nursing Press, New York

Fraser M 1996 Conceptual nursing in practice: a research-based approach, 2nd edn. Chapman and Hall, London

Greyson B 1993 Varieties of near death experience. Psychiatry 56(Nov.): 390–399

Greyson B, Evans Bush N 1992 Distressing near death experiences. Psychiatry 55(Feb.):95–109

Kellehear A 1993 Culture, biology and the near death experience: a reappraisal. The Journal of Nervous and Mental Disease 181(3):148–156

Maeve M 1998 Weaving a fabric of meaning: how nurses live with suffering and death. Journal of Advanced Nursing 27:1136–1142

Mallett J, Bailey C 1996 The Royal Marsden NHS Trust manual of clinical nursing procedures, 4th edn. Blackwell Science, Oxford, ch 24, pp. 334–338

Marks-Maran D 1997 In: Marks-Maran D, Rose P (eds) Reconstructing nursing. Beyond art and science. Baillière Tindall, London, ch 5, pp. 92–108

Morse J 1991 Negotiating commitment and involvement in the nurse patient relationship. Journal of Advanced Nursing 16:455–468

Morse M 1994 Near death experiences of children. Journal of Paediatric Oncology Nursing 11(4):139–144

Morse J, Bottorph J, Neander W, Solberg S 1991 Comparative analysis of conceptualizations and theories of caring. Image 23(2):119–126

Murphy D, Finucane T 1993 New do-not-resuscitate policies: a first step in cost control. Archives of Internal Medicine 153:1641–1648

Neuberger J 1987 Caring for dying people of different faiths. Austen Cornish, London

Page S, Meerabeau L 1996 Nurses' accounts of cardiopulmonary resuscitation. Journal of Advanced Nursing 24:317–325

Radwin L 1996 Knowing the patient: a review of research on an emerging concept. Journal of Advanced Nursing 23:1142–1146

Richardson G, Maynard A 1995 Fewer doctors? More nurses? A review of the knowledge base of doctor–nurse substitution, Discussion Paper 135. University of York, York

Roach S 1984 Caring: the human mode of being. Implications for nursing. Faculty of Nursing, Toronto

Roper N, Logan W, Tierney A 1996 The elements of nursing: a model for nursing based on a model for living, 4th edn. Churchill Livingstone, Edinburgh

Rose P, Parker D 1994 Nursing: an integration of art and science within the experience of the practitioner. Journal of Advanced Nursing 20: 1004–1010

Sabom M 1982 Recollections of death: a medical investigation. Harper and Row, London

Schön D 1991 The reflective practitioner. Avebury, Aldershot

UKCC 1992a Code of professional conduct, 3rd edn. UKCC, London

UKCC 1992b The scope of professional practice. UKCC, London

Vintner M 1994 An insight into the afterlife? Professional Nurse 10(3): 171–173

Watson J 1988 Nursing: human science and human care. National League for Nursing, New York

Watson J 1990 Caring knowledge and informed passion. Advances in Nursing Science 13(1):15–24

Watson J (ed.) 1994 Applying the art and science of human caring. National League for Nursing Press, New York

Watson S 1991 An analysis of the concept of experience. Journal of Advanced Nursing 16:1117–1121

Wright B 1996 Sudden death: a research base for practice, 2nd edn. Churchill Livingstone, Edinburgh

Care of relatives during resuscitation attempts

Sue Adams

■ CONTENTS

INTRODUCTION

'They also serve, who only stand and waite'

J. Milton 1608–1674 (On His Blindness)

Other contributors to this book have considered the legal and ethical issues, as well as the activities, processes and procedures of resuscitation. I will take you outside the arena of activity, beyond the white coats and frantic movements, to where friends or loved ones stand in a special place or a side-room off the main thoroughfare, disconnected from events, often finding themselves in silence.

The people who await your arrival could be sons or daughters, brothers or sisters, parents or partners, or anyone else who is related or connected to your patient. In accident and emergency (A&E) departments, they could be passers-by who have become involved in the incident leading to the patient's admission. They will need you to help them make sense of what is happening: in the future they may remember only fragments of what is happening but now they are looking to you to provide them with support.

This chapter aims to discuss some of the issues concerning the care of relatives. (For convenience, the term relative is used throughout to indicate the next of kin, partner or significant other designated by the patient.) You may already have many of the skills required to help your patient's relatives through this difficult time and so I have included reflection points that may be useful in the further development of these skills. This chapter also offers some guidelines and suggestions that you need to consider if you are to meet this challenge and become more effective in the support of the friends and families of patients who require cardiopulmonary resuscitation (CPR).

IDENTIFY WHO IS PRESENT AND WHY THEY ARE THERE

You need to begin by introducing yourself, giving both your name and your position. You also need to learn names of the people present and establish their relationship to the patient. This basic introduction will allow you time to consider your approach, to observe the behaviour of the people there and to open the lines of communication. They need to understand that your role is to provide them with the information and support that they need. This initial period can also help the individuals to gain some sense of reality in an otherwise confusing time.

If they are non-English speakers, you will need to identify their language and assess their ability to understand what you say. You should also try to assess any cultural and spiritual differences, which may give rise to conflicting expectations.

If there is a group, it may be possible to identify who is the dominant member, but note that they may not necessarily be the person who is closest to the patient, nor can they speak for the others.

You need to make eye contact with the individual you are addressing and to focus on them. You should try to find out when they last saw their relative. As a way of supporting a group, identify an individual who appears less distraught and link them with the most distressed. You should give them the information you have. You may need to repeat this more than once. It is helpful to provide access to a telephone, so that they can contact other relatives.

■ REFLECTION POINT 5.1

What is your fear of dealing with relatives and loved ones during this time?

- not knowing what to say
- saying too much
- saying too little
- not wanting to begin to feel what they are feeling
- saying the wrong thing.

Try to articulate your fears and discuss them with a colleague/preceptor/mentor at a quiet time.

Consider yourself in the position of the relatives. How would you wish to be approached?

WHAT SHOULD I SAY AND HOW SHOULD I SAY IT?

When speaking to relatives always use language that is:

- Simple (free of hospital abbreviations and technical detail)
- Honest (give an accurate and truthful account of what has happened)
- Unambiguous (free of euphemisms)
- Direct (get straight to the point).

The relatives should be told the truth about the events leading up to the arrest and what is currently happening. The language used should be comprehensible and clear: phrases such as 'He/she is poorly' mean nothing. Try to use more direct statements such as 'he/she is not breathing on their own', or 'his/her heart has stopped'. Avoid expressions such as 'they're working on him/her' – it makes the patient sound like a construction site. Greater clarity and sensitivity is provided by giving information such as 'the doctors are giving him/her drugs to improve the activity of their heart' or 'we are having to use equipment to breathe for him/her'.

HOW DO PEOPLE REACT?

The greater the emotional attachment and investment a person has in your patient the greater the feelings engendered. If the relatives were present when the loved one collapsed, they may be feeling fearful (Murray Parkes 1996). They may experience physiological symptoms such as dry mouth, urgency of micturition or of defaecation as a response to these feelings. They may appear pale whatever their original skin tone. They may shake, sometimes uncontrollably, or profess to feel cold. Anxiety is expressed in many ways, some of which may not be the way of your own culture. It may be difficult for you to appreciate that their means of expression is important to them. Some responses can be very loud and vocal, almost to the point of hysteria. The opposite reaction, which can be equally unnerving, is that of complete silence with no apparent desire to communicate with you. Individuals may cease to respond to you at all, and become closed-off in a safer inner world that may still hold for them a more secure previous reality. To accept you is to accept as fact the threat to that world bought about by the collapse and possible loss of their loved one.

You may need to repeat the information you have given several times to help these individuals accept what is happening. If they are on their own, you will need to keep your absences from them brief. Your responses should be nonjudgemental and supportive. Relatives experience both hope and despair when faced with the uncertain outcome of a resuscitation attempt. You need to help them accept that the outcome cannot be predicted. Note that most patients who are resuscitated do not survive (see chapter 8) and so it is wise to prepare them for the possibility that their loved one may die. This is one of the rare occasions when it is a pleasure to be proved wrong.

DO NOT GIVE UP YOUR ATTEMPTS TO COMMUNICATE

If you found barriers to communication when first you approached the relatives, you need to identify the cause and seek a remedy. If, for example the family do not speak English well enough to understand what you are saying, you will need to find a translator. Most hospitals have list of translators upon whom they can call in such situations. You may also need to consider getting additional help if the relatives and friends are visually or hearing impaired or have learning difficulties.

It is vital that relatives are kept informed of the situation, and this can take up a lot of additional time. During a resuscitation attempt, your first priority is the immediate physical needs of the patient (see chapter 4). Relatives are aware of this and would rather you devote your attention to your role in the resuscitation attempt. They will understand that you have very little time to spare during the resuscitation attempt. However, for nurses, the support of relatives is also part of our role and this can create conflicting demands on your time and attention (see chapter 4). It is generally best to explain openly why you cannot spare the time immediately but that you will try to keep them informed about what is happening as often as you can. The relatives need to be reassured that you will not forget them and that you will bring them to see their loved one as soon as possible.

WHAT IF RELATIVES WANT TO BE PRESENT DURING THE RESUSCITATION?

You need to explore this question with medical and nursing colleagues to prepare for this before a relative first makes this request. It is not appropriate to ask the team during an arrest situation if relatives can be present, as the answer will probably be an emphatic no. However, there is an increasing expectation between both staff and relatives that witnessed resuscitation should be allowed and even encouraged. There is now a body of published literature on the presence of relatives at resuscitation attempts. Although initially this was based on anecdotal evidence, recent research is more rigorous in its methodology and analysis. While many of the studies used numerically small samples and varying lengths of time over which the data was collected, there is a solid consistency in their findings that is strongly supportive of witnessed resuscitation (Doyle *et al.* 1987, Hanson & Strawser 1992, Adams *et al.* 1994, Connors 1996, Mitchell & Lynch 1997, Morgan 1997, Timmerman 1997, van der Woning 1997, Barratt & Wallis 1998, Ellison 1998, Robinson *et al.* 1998). There appears to be a less prolonged bereavement period and a quicker acceptance of the death of their relative or loved one. Interestingly, those patients that survive and know that a family member was present report feeling comforted by that knowledge. It is more common for parents to remain with their children at this time than for adult patients to have a loved one with them while being resuscitated. More centres within the UK (predominantly accident units) do provide the relatives with the vital support needed for this to occur. A number of accident units also ask relatives if they would like to be present (with support) during this time. Three things are essential before initiating witnessed resuscitation.

1. Find out how your clinical colleagues feel about the issue.
2. Obtain their consent and cooperation.
3. Ensure that someone is available whose only role is the support of the witness.

Effective support for witnesses of resuscitation attempts requires someone who is experienced in caring for relatives at this time. They should also have an in-depth understanding of resuscitation, its aetiology, manifestations, its treatment algorithms and all the associated interventions so that the situation can be explained simply but fully as it progresses.

LISTENING TO THE RELATIVES

In order for you to have a broad perspective of the needs of the people to whom you are speaking, a subtle yet dynamic use of various listening skills should be employed.

Silence

Do not be afraid of silence. It can be difficult to sit with a group of people and say nothing, and although you may find yourself feeling that you have to fill in the conversational space, this is best avoided. Sympathy can be conveyed without using words. Observe nonverbal signs from the individuals that they may wish to speak, and take your cue from them.

Passive listening

Passive listening is said to occur when listening allows for assimilation of information without any outward signs that this is occurring (Hargie *et al.* 1994). There may be situations in which listening passively allows relatives and friends to converse and to share anxieties without feeling that you need to become actively involved. The subtleties of family relationships and emotional partnerships are often hinted at during these moments. The ability to identify potentially contentious areas may allow you to avoid detrimental and upsetting confrontations. An example of this, which is increasingly common, is when first, second or even third spouses and/or partners may be present, leading to acrimonious meetings in corridors while the patient is being resuscitated. The ability to anticipate and defuse this unpleasant situation is aided by the use of passive listening.

Active listening

Active listening is said to occur when outward signs or behaviours are demonstrated to indicate that attention is being paid to the individual who is speaking. These signs and behaviours can be verbal or nonverbal. Their impact is varied and wide-ranging. At the very least, they provide 'live' commas and full stops so that the speaker can take account of what they themselves are saying and possibly change direction in the meaning or explanation of the meaning. Their greatest impact is that of conveying a sensitive empathy to the speaker from you the listener (Hargie *et al.* 1994), thus paving the way for a supportive relationship to develop. This relationship may be transitory but is essential for the duration of the resuscitation attempt and for the immediate aftercare of relatives.

INFORMING RELATIVES WHO ARE NOT PRESENT

Whether you work in a ward, critical care area or an accident unit, there may be a need for you to make contact with absent relatives, friends or partners. During the assessment/admission process, a contact person must be identified. This might not be your patient's next of kin, but should be someone to whom they would give their trust to act for them. You may have to ask them who they would wish called should there be an emergency. This question should be asked with some subtlety and tact to avoid causing them unnecessary worry.

If no contact person is identified, you will need to search property/possessions in order to establish possible addresses or telephone numbers. If that fails, then help from the local police force can be sought. They may be able to visit the home and/or follow up addresses. They may also be able to obtain information from neighbours about next of kin or other people close to your patient.

Even if you have contact numbers, there may still be other problems. If the relatives or friends live nearby, then information can be given to indicate the seriousness of the situation and the need for their presence explained. However, if they are at a distance or overseas, you and your colleagues will have to make a decision regarding the level and detail of the information that should be provided. The usual procedure is not to give information over the telephone; however, each case must be judged individually. I know of occasions when relatives have been given too little information and have travelled great distances in the mistaken belief that they would arrive before the death of their loved ones. The distress this causes can only be imagined.

As a junior staff nurse, I was instructed not to give information over the phone until the person I was talking to had someone with them. However, this unnecessary delay and prevarication merely created extra problems in an already difficult situation and served only to extend the period of worry.

When giving information during a telephone conversation, consider the following points:

- Find out to whom you are speaking
- State who you are and what your designation/position is
- Give the location of their relative, i.e. clinic/surgery/ward/ hospital
- Confirm the relationship or connection the person on the phone has with your patient
- Tell them what has happened and what is happening now
- Ask them to consider whether they wish to come to the ward or patient's bedside
- If they are not sure, give them a phone number and suggest they think about it
- Tell them that you will contact them with regular updates on the patient's progress as circumstances allow
- Ask for the contact numbers of close friends or other family members who live nearby who might be prepared to come to the hospital and provide a family link at the bedside
- Be prepared to give the name of another member of staff if you are about to go off shift
- Be direct
- Keep the language simple and clear and avoid euphemisms.

■ REFLECTION POINT 5.2

Discuss with family and friends how they would expect to be informed if you or another member of your family were to be taken seriously ill.

WHAT DO I SAY IF RELATIVES ASK IF THE PATIENT IS GOING TO DIE?

Once a patient has suffered a cardio-respiratory arrest, there is always a possibility that they may die, and you should say so. Temper this with information about what is being done to prevent death occurring; however, engendering false hope is cruel. You need to ensure that they appreciate the seriousness of the situation. Note that following resuscitation, successful outcomes in the long term are the exception (see chapter 8).

On a number of occasions I have let relatives or loved ones of my patient know that despite drugs and support to breathe, the patient is not responding and that a recovery is unlikely. If then asked if this means death is going to ensue, my reply has been 'yes if no change occurs', or 'it's very likely, because they are not responding to treatment'. If the patient's condition has then improved, it has been a pleasure to tell relatives of the reversal of events. This does have to be accompanied by a warning of a possible return to the critical state, but relatives generally appreciate being informed of what is happening.

WHAT HAPPENS WHEN THE RESUSCITATION ATTEMPT IS SUCCESSFUL?

The relatives will need to know what the sequence of events will be following this outcome. The patient will be stabilized and possibly transferred to an intensive care unit. It should be explained that close observation will be required as the patient's condition is still very serious and that many patients arrest again in the immediate post-resuscitation period.

If the patient is to be transferred, the relatives will need to know where they are going and whether they can accompany them. They may wish to see their relative before the transfer and this you should facilitate as quickly as possible so that the transfer is not delayed. They will need to know about any equipment being used and its purpose, e.g. chest drains, central intravenous lines, endotracheal tubes, ventilation equipment. You need to know why the patient has these in place and when discussing these interventions you need to be able to translate clinical and technical terminology into clear, simple English. You will therefore need to have a comprehensive knowledge and understanding of all the interventions that may have been used in a resuscitation attempt (see chapters 6, 7, 9 and 10).

■ REFLECTION POINT 5.3

As part of your ongoing personal and professional development, you might consider using a 'Critical Incident' technique to explore an experience of resuscitation. This would enable you to consider the event at a time when there are few distractions. You might feel that it would be helpful to discuss your perception of the event with a senior colleague, especially your method of dealing with relatives. The completed reflection could then be inserted into your professional portfolio (UKCC 1997).
An example of the technique is as follows (after Johns 1994):

• Write a description of the experience.
• In what way was this incident critical?
• What were your concerns at the time?
• What were you thinking about as the incident was taking place?
• What were your feelings during and after the incident?
• Did you find anything particularly demanding about the incident and if so why?
• Did you find anything satisfying about the incident? Why?

In identifying what you have learned from the experience, consider Carper's (1978) 'Ways of Knowing':

Aesthetics – what were you trying to achieve? Why did you respond as you did? What were the consequences for those involved?

Empirics – what knowledge did you use, and was it sufficient in depth and breadth? If you are dissatisfied with your level of knowledge, what can you do to improve it?

Ethics – did your behaviour and actions fit with your beliefs? If not, where was the discrepancy?

Personal – having recognized your feelings during this experience, how could you see yourself acting in a similarly stressful situation? Can you link this experience with any other that you have had in your life?

A major consideration during any experience must be your own personal safety, physically, mentally, spiritually and professionally:

- Have you identified ways in which you can gain effective support from family, friends and colleagues? (Boud *et al.* 1985)
- If there has been a successful outcome, consider following up the patient and their family, and their perspective on the whole event.

While this might not be practical for each resuscitation you are involved in, there is certainly a place for you to include the family's experience alongside your own in the initial period of your new role.

WHAT IF THE RESUSCITATION IS UNSUCCESSFUL?

If you have maintained contact with the relatives or friends of the patient throughout resuscitation, then you should have prepared them for this. Local policies will usually determine who should inform them of the death. This may be the senior member of the medical staff or a senior nurse. If you have been involved with the relatives, you should try to continue the contact you have established and maintain the continuity of their care by accompanying the person who is designated the task. The trust that you have engendered will help the relatives to feel that they have an advocate during this time.

There is a wide range of possible reactions to the news. Generally, there is a peaceful but emotional response; it may be a silent one. Occasionally, however, there may be physical violence. Colleagues have informed me of punches being thrown and equipment broken, therefore, you need to be prepared for this possibility. Your skills in observing the nonverbal cues will be essential in predicting extreme reactions and in preparing yourself to deal with them. Most people will send out signals (such as increasing inability to stay still, inability to articulate their anger and frustration or the clenching of fists and jaw) before finally erupting. You may also be aware of evidence of substance abuse (such as drugs or alcohol) in the people you are dealing with and this increases the possibility of violence as part of their response to this difficult situation. Violence is rare in a ward situation but more common in A&E departments.

If the relatives or loved ones have been present during the resuscitation attempt they will need comfort and support to remain near while the usual 'tidying and clearing up' occurs. This should be done as unobtrusively and sensitively as possible.

Do not hurry the communication process

Time needs to be given for the news of death to be assimilated. If you have been with the relatives throughout you will be able to offer them the opportunity to be with your patient and to begin the grieving process. They may want time to make physical contact (especially while the body is still warm). The type of contact can range from holding and kissing the hands to lying alongside the body. In children, the usual contact is holding or a cuddle. Your help will be needed as very few people will have ever dealt with a dead body, and there are many myths about death and dead bodies. It is almost as if the body becomes more fragile. In the situation of a serocompromised patient you will need to balance the safety needs of both staff and relatives, allowing grief to be expressed through contact yet minimizing the dangers of leaking body fluids.

Spiritual and religious considerations

It is at times like these that people often turn to their religious and spiritual beliefs to provide reasons for what has happened. For some, this provides comfort, for others who have no or little religious faith comfort may have to be found from other sources. The hospital chaplain can provide nondenominational spiritual and practical support to both relatives and staff. They can also help contact ministers of other religions if the family does not have this information and wishes to speak with a minister of their own faith.

There may be cultural and religious observances that should be observed at this time, as a mark of respect for your patient and in support of the grieving family. You should ensure that your knowledge of the community you serve includes this kind of cultural information.

Special circumstances

You may be present, when in certain circumstances, permission may be sought for the harvesting of organs, or relatives may request that organs be donated. In this event, the local transplant coordinator should be contacted for information and advice. The body may be moved to intensive care for ventilation or may be sent to the mortuary and organs taken later.

A post mortem may be necessary to identify cause of death, and relatives may find this upsetting. The patient may have been the victim of violence and be the subject of police enquiries. In these situations, you may have to consider legal issues if further investigation into the circumstances of the death is likely to follow. It is not unknown for evidence to be lost due to tampering with a body by relatives. You may need to explain this to the relatives, should they wish to be alone with the body in this situation. In these rare circumstances, tact is essential, as is patience. Sometimes, anger may be expressed in outright rejection of these procedures. You will need to listen to the responses and be prepared to explain the necessity and rationales for these procedures.

Preparing the body for viewing

If the relatives wish to view the body, it is important that any remaining evidence of the interventions used during the resuscitation attempt should be explained. Clinical waste and body fluids should be removed and the area made clean. Equipment that may be needed again for another patient should be taken away. However, it is not essential to display the body as if in a funeral parlour. You will have explained what has occurred and they will expect to see evidence of that level of activity.

The usual requirements are for limbs to be straightened, eyes closed and for clean linen to be used to cover the body in order to maintain the patient's dignity in death. Any relevant local protocols, practices or policies should be followed before the viewing takes place. A nurse should accompany the relatives to view the body so that support may be given as needed, and any questions that they might have can be answered. In most situations, a few moments alone with the deceased allow relatives to say their farewells as an important stage of the grieving process.

There has been a custom for nurses to leave the body for a period after death has occurred and before last offices are performed. This perhaps provides time for the nursing staff to restore order and calm before giving their patient their last gentle care. After a resuscitation attempt there is a need to consider quietly the event that has just occurred and reflect upon its professional and human consequences (see chapter 4). Demands upon nursing time and bed space are now so great that we have little time for this kind of activity; however, it is important to obtain a perspective on what has happened. There is a commonly held belief that it is during the hour following death that the soul leaves the body, and I, like many other nurses, continue to talk to my patient at this time, partly to make my own farewells and partly because I do not know at what point cognitive awareness is lost. I did not always do this, especially when I was younger as I felt I might be mocked or scorned. I now believe that it helps to break the ties gently between you and the individual you have nursed during the final moments of their life.

In the past, nurses were expected to remain detached and not to show any emotional reaction to their patient's death, especially after unsuccessful resuscitation attempts. When they did so, it was deemed unprofessional. However, I have heard relatives say that they were comforted by a nurse who shed tears for their loved one, because it indicated to them that the nurse, although not part of the family, genuinely cared. You may feel very upset by the death of a patient, but the relatives need your professional support and their needs should be uppermost in your mind. If you have been deeply affected by the resuscitation attempt and the death of the patient, you need to ensure that your own emotional and professional needs are met. Make use of any available mentoring/preceptorship/clinical supervision schemes within your clinical area. If there are none, explore the possibility of setting up this kind of professional support.

Relatives may wish to help in the final care given before the body is removed to the mortuary. This is something that you should discuss beforehand with your colleagues. I have performed 'Last Offices' with the relative of the patient and found it moving because it represents a shared respect and valuing of the individual who has died.

Accompanying the body and relatives to the mortuary

In certain circumstances, you may be required to accompany relatives to the mortuary to view the body. It is important that you go on a 'reconnaissance' long before you need to go with relatives. The last thing that relatives need is for a nurse to get them lost in a labyrinth of hospital corridors. You will need to check the layout and establish whether it is a sympathetic environment. Is there any recognition of the needs of grieving relatives to have a quiet area away from the clinical appearance of a mortuary? If not, then you may need to consider giving a warning to that effect. It is important to find out what may have to be done by the mortuary technicians before the body is ready for viewing. This is especially true if the patient was disfigured in any way by trauma, surgery before the arrest occurred or by medical intervention during the resuscitation attempt. You may need to remain with relatives while they make their farewells and then accompany their return to the ward/unit area since they will be unlikely to remember the route taken.

In some care areas, babies may be carried to the mortuary by nursing staff. Children may be taken in a white coffin or carried by their parents. You should be aware of any particular practices in your own work area, but you also need to be receptive to the expressed needs of the parents during this time.

CONCLUSION

Resuscitation is one of the most demanding situations faced by all health professionals involved, and by the patients and their relatives. It is a traumatic event and, as such, will always provoke extremes of anxiety and emotion. Your role will be to reduce the level of anxiety experienced and thus enable relatives to begin to deal with the emotional legacy of the experience. You will already have many of the skills required to help your patients and their relatives through this difficult time. The most important element in your approach will be your honesty in your responses to them at all stages of the resuscitation process.

You too will need to deal with the legacy of this experience. By reflecting on the event with a trusted, more experienced colleague, you will be able to learn from it, expand your understanding of your own abilities and develop confidence in your skills in dealing with relatives in these intense situations.

■ **REFLECTION POINT 5.4**   POINTS TO REMEMBER

The most important elements in the nursing care of distressed relatives are:

- Honesty in your responses at all stages of the resuscitation process
- Good communication skills to provide full and frequent information
- Respect for the feelings of the patient and their relatives
- Respect for the spiritual beliefs of the patient and their relatives.

REFERENCES

Adams S, Whitlock M, Higgs R, Bloomfield P, Basket P J F 1994 Should relatives be allowed to watch resuscitation? British Medical Journal 308: 1687–1692

Barratt F, Wallis D N 1998 Relatives in the resuscitation room: their point of view. Journal of Accident and Emergency Medicine 15:109–111

Benner P, Wrubel J 1989 The primacy of caring. Addison Wesley, Menlo Park

Boud D, Keogh R, Walker D (eds) 1985 Reflection: turning experience into learning. Kogan Page, London

Carper B A 1978 Fundamental patterns of knowing in nursing. Advances in Nursing Science 1(1):13–23

Connors T 1996 Should relatives be allowed in the resuscitation room? Nursing Standard 10(44):42–44

Doyle C J, Post H, Burney R E et al. 1987 Family participation during resuscitation: an option. Annals of Emergency Medicine 16(6):673–675

Ellison G 1998 Witnessed resuscitation: The relatives' experience. Emergency Nurse Dec–Jan 5(8):27–29

Hanson C, Strawser D 1992 Family presence during cardiopulmonary resuscitation: Foote Hospital Emergency Department's nine-year perspective. Journal of Emergency Nursing 18(2):104–106

Hargie O, Saunders C, Dickson D (1994) Social skills in interpersonal communication, 3rd edn. Routledge, London

Johns C C 1994 Guided reflection. In: Palmer A, Burns S, Bulman C (eds) Reflective practice in nursing. Blackwell Scientific, Oxford

Mitchell A H, Lynch M B 1997 Should relatives be allowed into the resuscitation room? Journal of Accident Emergency Medicine 14:366–369

Morgan J 1997 Introducing witnessed resuscitation in A & E. Emergency Nurse 13, Vol. 5(2):13–18

Murray Parkes C M 1996 Bereavement, 3rd edn. Penguin Books, West Drayton

Robinson S M, Mackenzie-Ross S, Campbell Hewson G L, Egleston C V, Prevost A T 1998 Psychological effect of witnessed resuscitation on bereaved relatives. Lancet 352(9128):614–617

Timmerman S 1997 High touch in high tech: The presence of friends during resuscitation efforts. Scholarly Inquiry for Nursing Practice: an International Journal 11(2):153–167

UKCC 1997 Prep and you. UKCC, London

van der Woning M 1997 Should relatives be invited to witness a resuscitation attempt? Accident & Emergency Nursing 5:215–218

FURTHER READING

Bailey R D 1985 Coping with stress in caring. Blackwell Publications, Oxford
Edlich R F, Kubler-Ross E 1992 On death and dying in the emergency room. Journal of Emergency Medicine 10:225–229
McLauchlan C 1996 Should relatives witness resuscitation? Resuscitation Council (UK), London

Basic life support

Di Smith

INTRODUCTION

All nurses, whatever their role, speciality or practice context, must be able to carry out basic life support (BLS) because, according to our Professional Code of Conduct (UKCC 1992) we must ensure that no act or omission on our part is detrimental to patients or clients. The public has a right to expect that all nurses, including those who do not have direct patient contact, but whose employment requires registration with the UKCC, such as academics and managers, should be able to carry out BLS. Cardiorespiratory arrest can occur at any time and at any place: it can happen to patients, colleagues, family, friends or strangers and it can take place anywhere. You never know where or when you might become involved in the attempt to save a life. This chapter aims to explain the BLS algorithm and enhance your theoretical knowledge of its principles and application. Obviously, this chapter is no substitute for 'hands-on' skill development, so it is strongly recommended that, after reading this chapter, you should practice your skills on a manikin under the supervision of a trainer. Local voluntary organizations (see chapter 13) or your local resuscitation training officer offer this kind of skills training to health service employees and the general public. In this chapter, I describe briefly the background to the BLS algorithm and define BLS. I include a brief discussion of conditions that may predispose to cardiac arrest and the role of the nurse in the assessment and observation of those who are at risk. The BLS guidelines will then be given with discussion of their use in both the hospital setting and in out-of-hospital resuscitation attempts. Please refer to chapter 13 for further discussion of resuscitation in the community setting.

In 1997, the BLS working group for the International Liaison Committee on Resuscitation (ILCOR) produced advisory statements for the single rescuer adult life support. These statements represented the consensus view of the world's major resuscitation organizations (Handley *et al.* 1997). In producing the guidelines, the BLS groups of the European Resuscitation Council (ERC) studied the advisory statements and reviewed feedback on their use during 1997 from a number of training organizations in Europe (Bossaert 1998). The process of the development of the advisory statements involved identification of major and minor differences that existed between the BLS guidelines of the American Heart Association (1992) and the working party of the European Resuscitation Council (1992). A consensus was reached and preparation of the final sequence of actions was published in 1997 at the ERC conference at Brighton, UK, and ratified in 1998 in Copenhagen, Denmark. The modifications that were made to the BLS template were not intended to restrict national organizations, or to prevent them from making changes to the template when valid concerns or research studies support it. The central concern was to make the guidelines as simple as possible, to simplify training and to ensure uniformity across the world (Bossaert 1998).

BLS means that no equipment is used for rescue breathing; when a simple airway or facemask for mouth to mask resuscitation is used, this is referred to as BLS with airway adjunct (Resuscitation Council (UK) 1998). The purpose of BLS is to maintain adequate ventilation and circulation until the cause of the arrest is identified and advanced life support (ALS) protocols instigated. It is seen as a 'holding operation', although there are occasions when it may reverse the cause, e.g. in respiratory arrest (Bossaert 1998).

PATIENTS AT RISK

Cardiopulmonary arrest is defined as the cessation of breathing and cardiac output and is often referred to as cardiac arrest in hospital. If rescue measures are commenced to breathe for the victim (rescue breathing) and chest compressions instigated, the term cardiopulmonary resuscitation is used. This secures adequate oxygenation and cardiac output until the underlying cause can be treated.

If a patient stops breathing but still has a cardiac output (pulse can be palpated), this is referred to as respiratory arrest.

It is important that nurses are familiar with the variety of conditions that may predispose a patient to developing cardiopulmonary arrest or respiratory arrest. Regardless of the specialist area in which the patient may be nursed, there are a number of conditions that have a high risk for cardiac and/or respiratory arrest.

Patients in medical wards suffering from pathologies such as chronic obstructive airways disease (COAD) and asthma are predisposed to developing respiratory distress and arrest. What may not be so obvious is the development of a tension pneumothorax (see Case history 6.1). Patients developing respiratory arrest are also at risk of developing bradycardia

---

Case history 6.1

A patient had become very distressed following administration of his nebulized drugs. He became cyanotic very rapidly and quickly collapsed with what appeared to be a seizure. BLS was commenced and a cardiac monitor attached. The monitor showed electrical activity that was similar to sinus rhythm leading to the diagnosis of electrical mechanical dissociation (EMD; see chapter 7). It was noted, on ventilating the patient, that there was lack of chest movement on the left side. The on-call anaesthetist quickly diagnosed tension pneumothorax and a large-bore needle was inserted in the second intercostal space in the left mid-clavicular line. As the pressure was relieved, a hissing sound was heard and cardiac output returned.

---

followed by asystole, as a result of hypoxia. Hence, there is a need to assess breathing and begin ventilating the patient as a priority in order to maintain cardiac activity.

Myocardial infarction (MI) is the most obvious condition with which cardiac arrest is associated. Nurses caring for these patients should also be aware of the peri-arrest rhythms that could deteriorate into ventricular fibrillation (VF) or pulseless ventricular tachycardia (VT) (see chapter 7). These are not the only considerations for MI sufferers: other potential complications include cardiac tamponade and acute heart failure, which could result in EMD.

In surgical wards, patients are at risk of hypovolaemia, which may follow surgery or trauma. Fluid overload can also cause heart failure and respiratory failure due to pulmonary oedema, which may deteriorate to the point of cardiorespiratory arrest. Accurate and frequent recordings of fluid intake and output are essential tools in the assessment of fluid balance and a falling urine output/oliguria (urine output < 30 mL/h for more than 2 h) or an increasingly positive balance should be reported to medical staff. Deep-vein thrombosis, leading to pulmonary embolism is a recognized complication of bed rest in both medical and surgical patients. Adverse drug reactions and electrolyte disturbances are also risk factors for cardiorespiratory arrest (see chapter 7, Tables 7.1 and 7.2), which may occur in medical or surgical patients. Many hospital patients are elderly and suffer from multiple pathologies that may complicate the condition for which they were admitted.

The role of the ward nurse is pivotal in the prevention of cardiorespiratory arrest in hospital patients. The nurse should be skilled in the physical assessment of patients and have a sound theoretical knowledge base for practice, which ensures the intelligent interpretation of assessment data. This enables the nurse to identify severely ill patients and to instigate frequent observation of their vital signs and symptoms. If the nurse diagnoses that the patient's condition is deteriorating, medical support can be summoned and, through early medical intervention, cardiorespiratory arrest may be prevented. Nurses must recognize the vital part they play in observing their patients and preventing cardiorespiratory arrest in hospitals.

RECOGNIZING THE SIGNS OF CARDIOPULMONARY ARREST

Whatever the predisposing factors, the signs of cardiac arrest will be the same. The patient will collapse, sometimes this may be witnessed and in hospitals, the ALS algorithm (see chapter 7) should be followed as soon as possible. Early defibrillation (if appropriate) should be the priority if it is available (see chapter 10). The patient may appear to be having a seizure (an experience that I have witnessed while working in coronary care with patients who have developed VF). Changes in the patient's colour, i.e. the presence of cyanosis and/or pallor may also be observed. In all cases, breathing is either agonal or absent and there is no carotid pulse.

Cardiac arrest is very often perceived by nurses as a sudden occurrence; however, as already discussed, this is often not the case in hospitals. The sequence of actions to be taken on suspicion that a patient has had a cardiac arrest is given in Fig. 6.1, but it is advised that on approaching the patient the nurse should pay attention to their own safety. I recall an incident when a colleague ran over to a patient who had collapsed. On collapsing, the patient had knocked over his water jug and my colleague slipped on the water and hit her shin on the metal bar on the side of the bed. While there were no bones broken, the injury caused pain and discomfort for months following the event. This first measure of checking safety for the rescuer is especially important in out-of-hospital resuscitation. Hazards such as risk of drowning, electrocution or fire must be assessed before approach-

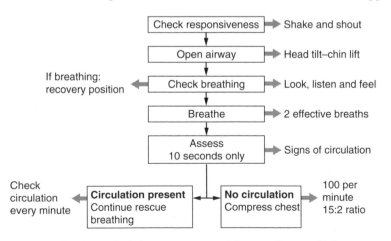

Fig. 6.1 Adult basic life support. Resuscitation Council (UK) 1998, reproduced with permission.

ing the victim. Rescuers have died trying to save others through disregard for their own safety. This not only increases the difficulties for the emergency services but also unnecessarily doubles the human tragedy.

CHECK RESPONSE

If cardiac arrest is suspected then it is recommended that the patient should be shaken gently on the shoulders and asked if he/she is all right (Resuscitation Council (UK) 1998). The purpose is to elicit a response in order to rule out other causes of collapse. At this point, the nurse or health professional should summon help by calling out for assistance or by using the emergency call bell. It is vital for the rescuer or nurse to get help as quickly as possible. The first link in the chain of survival is to gain access to the emergency services. In hospital, this is the emergency resuscitation team (also referred to as the crash team). The chance of survival is increased the sooner ALS is initiated (see chapters 7, 8 and 10). Improving the chances of survival from a cardiac arrest begins with early access. According to the 'Chain of Survival' (Fig. 6.2), the sooner the help is summoned the greater the chance of survival (Cummins *et al.* 1991).

If there is no response from the patient, the next action is to open the airway.

OPEN AIRWAY

The airway can be opened by using the head tilt–chin lift manoeuvre (Fig. 6.3). It is recommended, however, that before doing this, the mouth is opened and checked for anything that may fall into the oropharynx when the manoeuvre is applied (see Case history 6.2). When it is established that the airway is clear, the head tilt–chin lift manoeuvre will prevent the tongue from occluding the airway. If the patient is wearing well-fitted dentures that do not move away from the gums easily, then it is recommended that they be left in place.

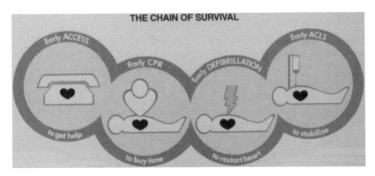

Fig. 6.2 Chain of Survival. Reproduced with the permission of Laerdal Medical Ltd, Orpington BR6 0HX, UK.

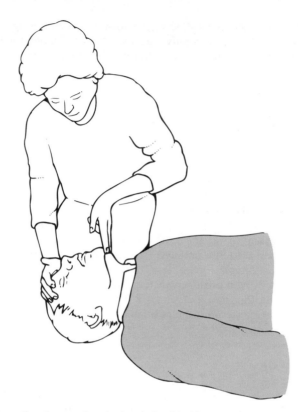

Fig. 6.3 Open the airway using the head tilt–chin lift manoeuvre.

Case history 6.2

A colleague had difficulty ventilating a patient who was found collapsed. BLS was commenced with the head tilt–chin lift manoeuvre and it was established that there was no breathing. Two rescue breaths were given, with difficulty. A carotid pulse check revealed no output and chest compressions were commenced. As there had been difficulty with the initial rescue breaths, the nurse managing the airway checked the mouth following the first five chest compressions. An obstruction at the back of the mouth could be seen and was quickly removed. It transpired that the patient had suffered a stroke while eating his lunch. The obstruction was a piece of chicken that had not been noticed on the initial assessment. The ventilations had forced the chicken back into the mouth of the patient where it was observed and duly removed.

It should be noted that this manoeuvre could be used in whatever position the patient is found. It is not necessary to lay the patient down first for this manoeuvre if they are sitting up when discovered. In some circumstances, e.g. where the patient has lost consciousness, the simple act of head tilt–chin lift will stop the tongue occluding the airway. If no breath sounds are heard then the next step of the sequence is followed.

CHECK BREATHING

Look, listen and feel for signs of breathing by looking at the chest while listening for breath sounds and feeling for any breath exhaled by the patient. This action will be made easier by the nurse bringing their cheek over the patient's mouth and nose (Fig. 6.4) and turning his/her face towards the patient's feet. It is recommended that this check be carried out for up to 10 s (Bossaert 1998). This is particularly appropriate for the novice nurse, although a more experienced nurse or health professional could make the diagnosis in less than 10 s, based on signs such as cyanosis, pallor of the skin and the stillness of the patient. There are occasions when the patient appears to be making a breathing effort. However, when listening and feeling for exhalations, the breaths cannot be heard or felt. This is known as agonal breathing and can be described as breathing effort (and in some cases hiccoughing) without breath sounds. If there is any doubt about the patient's ability to breath then the nurse or health professional should move on to the next step of BLS – breathing.

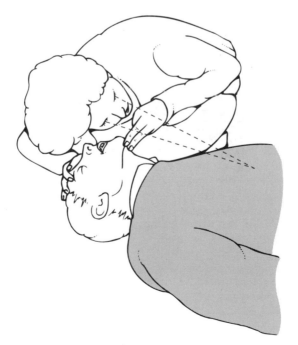

Fig. 6.4 Look, listen and feel for breath sounds.

At this point, if help has arrived, the other rescuer should call the ambulance and any other necessary emergency services. In hospital, the advanced resuscitation team should be called using the local emergency call system and any available resuscitation equipment collected. In the event that help has not arrived, then the nurse or rescuer will have to decide whether or not to leave the patient and go and summon help. In out-of-hospital situations, the decision must be made according to the estimated time it would take to obtain help. The patient should then be laid flat on their back (if not already doing so) and breathing commenced.

BREATHING

When cardiac arrest occurs in hospital, it is recommended by the Resuscitation Council (UK) (1998) that breathing for the patient should be with the use of adjuncts such as a pocket mask or the bag-valve mask unit (see chapter 9). If these resources are not available, then mouth-to-mouth resuscitation should be commenced. Two rescue breaths are given (Fig. 6.5) by opening the airway (Fig. 6.6) and blowing steadily into the mouth, ensuring a good seal around the mouth. The nurse should then look up at the chest to see the chest wall lowering (Fig. 6.7).

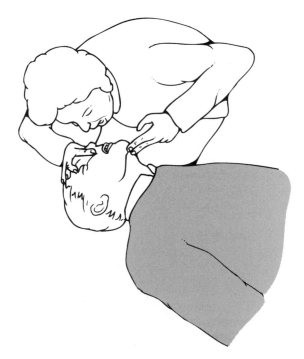

Fig. 6.5 Two rescue breaths are given by opening the airway.

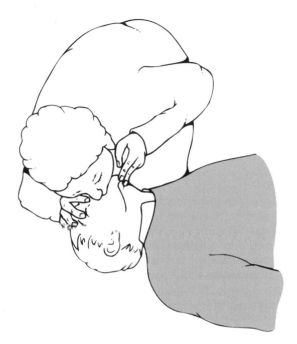

Fig. 6.6 Blow steadily into the mouth, ensuring a good seal around it.

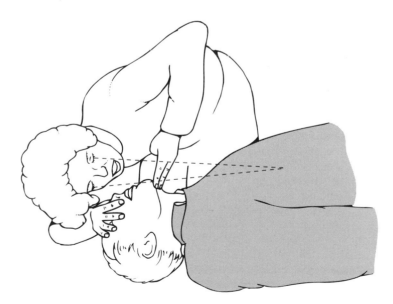

Fig. 6.7 Look up at the chest to see the chest wall lowering.

If difficulty is experienced in ventilating the patient, i.e. the chest does not appear to rise, and there is a feeling of resistance – likened to the feeling of resistance felt when blowing up a new balloon – then the airway should be checked and the head tilt–chin lift manoeuvre repeated. As soon as two successful breaths are made, the next step of the algorithm is to check the pulse. Even if there is no success in breathing for the patient, only five breathing attempts should be made and the assessment moved on to the next step in the algorithm (Resuscitation Council (UK) 1998).

Before the 1997 ILCOR statements were made, the volume of air required for each ventilation was given as 800–1200 mL, with each breath taking 1–15 s. The validity of the figures was questioned by the BLS advisory group (Bossaert 1998). Rescue breathing carries a high risk of gastric inflation, regurgitation of stomach content, followed by pulmonary aspiration. Studies by Baskett *et al.* (1996) showed that 400–500 mL is sufficient to give adequate ventilation in adult BLS because carbon dioxide production during cardiac arrest is very low. This recommendation overrides the previous guidelines and has resulted in the need to recalibrate existing resuscitation manikins. However, the recommendation is consistent with the accepted teaching practice that the tidal volume should be sufficient to cause the chest to rise (Bossaert 1998).

PULSE CHECK

Nurses who are familiar with the pre-1997 BLS guidelines will be aware that the time taken to check the carotid pulse has changed from 5 s to 10 s. An experienced nurse would probably carry this out at the same time as the breathing assessment. This change results from a number of studies undertaken to establish the efficacy of the carotid pulse check (Flesche *et al.* 1994, Eberle *et al.* 1996, Mather & O'Kelly 1996). These studies suggest that the time required to diagnose the presence or absence of carotid pulse is much greater than 5–10 s. Bahr *et al.* (1997) showed that 45% of carotid pulses might be identified as absent even when present. It should be considered however, that most of these studies used volunteers who were healthy rather than collapsed, cyanosed, hypotensive or vasoconstricted. In the light of these studies, the BLS advisory group recommended that the carotid pulse be de-emphasized and that attention should be paid to looking for signs of circulation, e.g. any movement. However, in hospital, the carotid pulse check is part of the ALS algorithm and is a skill that nurses should acquire. The pulse check should not exceed 10 s (Resuscitation Council (UK) 1998).

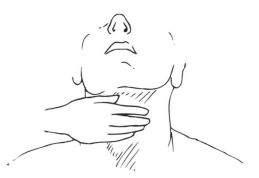

Fig. 6.8 Locating carotid pulse.

A technique to locate the carotid pulse is to extend the fingers and place the middle joint of the second finger gently on the patient's trachea (at the point of the larynx/Adam's apple; Fig. 6.8). The hand is then tilted so that the fingers press on the groove in the neck next to the trachea. It does not matter from which side the nurse approaches the patient to do this (the branches of the carotid arteries run up on either side of the trachea). This technique can be easily practised in order to become confident in locating the carotid pulse. Students and staff should check carotid pulses on a regular basis: checking the carotid pulse on a collapsed patient should not be the first occasion that the nurse has performed this skill.

If circulation is present, then rescue breathing is continued with each rescue breath taking 1.5–2 s for breathing and 3 s for expiration. This will give an approximate rate of 10 respirations per 40–60 s (Resuscitation Council (UK) 1998). The circulation is then checked every minute.

CHEST COMPRESSIONS

If circulation is absent, then chest compressions must be commenced. This produces a cardiac output by applying direct downward force and compression. The pressure in the thoracic cavity rises and blood is ejected via the aorta. The spring effect of the rib cage creates a rebound when the hands release the downward force and this results in a negative intrathoracic pressure, which draws venous blood into the heart. The correct position for chest compressions and procedure is given in Figure 6.9.

a

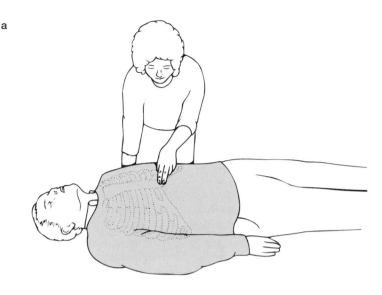

b

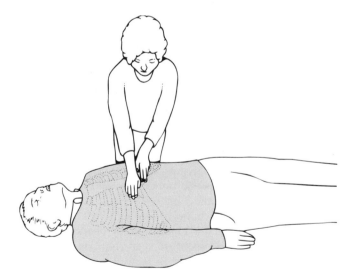

Fig. 6.9 Chest compressions. The correct position is located by sliding the fingers down the sternum or along the border of the lower ribs until the lower end of the sternum is found. The middle finger of one hand is placed on the end of the sternum and the index finger of the same hand next to it (a). The second hand is then placed next to the index finger of the first hand (b) and then the first hand placed on top (c). The fingers are interlocked and lifted in order to keep pressure off the ribs during compressions. It is important to ensure that the elbows are locked straight and that the shoulders of the nurse giving the compressions are directly over the chest (d).

c

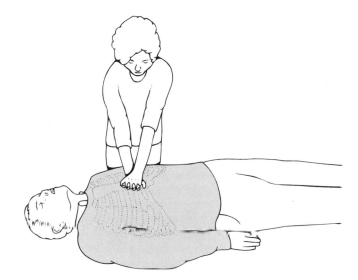

d

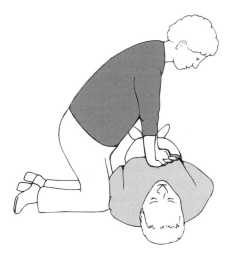

Fig. 6.9 contd This ensures that the force is applied vertically over the sternum, reducing the risk of fractured ribs. The sternum should be depressed by no more than about 4 cm. Fifteen compressions are delivered with two rescue breaths if the nurse is acting as a single rescuer. When a second nurse or rescuer is available to assist, and if the resuscitation team (or emergency services) has been alerted, then five compressions to one breath are given. The ratio of compressions is 100/min, which is approximately 15 compressions in 12 s.

PREGNANCY

When cardiac arrest occurs in pregnancy the patient and the fetus must be considered. If the patient is in the later stages of the pregnancy then consideration must be given to the venous return and cardiac output of the patient. Pressure on the inferior vena cava from the pregnant uterus can reduce the venous return and impair cardiac output. This can be relieved by placing pillows under the right side of the patient or moving and keeping the uterus to the left side manually (Resuscitation Council (UK) 1998). Chest compressions are then continued as described above, but they may be difficult owing to splinting of the diaphragm by the gravid uterus and breast hypertrophy.

With BLS underway and the emergency team alerted, other members of staff should then collect the resuscitation trolley or equipment. It is important that all nurses are familiar with the equipment in their clinical area. Some hospital wards have resuscitation trolleys that house all the equipment needed in an arrest situation (i.e. airway management equipment, oxygen, defibrillator, suction and emergency drugs). Other wards may have the equipment stored in one place but not on one trolley. It is the responsibility of the nurse to know what equipment is available, where it is kept and how to use it. The nurse should ensure that it is in working order, complete and ready to use. As a ward sister, one of the safety checks that I carried out following the hand-over period was checking that the resuscitation equipment was in order. This was a requirement for each shift and student nurses and new staff members were taught to carry out the check so that they could become familiar with the equipment.

When the equipment is at the bedside, the defibrillation monitor should be attached to the patient so that the rhythm can be identified (see chapter 7). The equipment required for advanced airway management (see chapter 9), should be placed near to the patient's head ready for use when the ALS team arrives. The emergency drugs can be laid out ready to use and the oxygen and suction (if not wall-mounted) prepared. However, the emphasis must be on BLS. While working as a sister in a medical unit I was required to attend cardiac arrests when holding the medical unit bleep. I can recall how frustrating it was to find, on arrival, that staff would be attending to the equipment but no BLS was being performed. This is still a problem that is reported anecdotally by colleagues and resuscitation training now places the emphasis on the importance of instigating and maintaining BLS. For further details of the nurse's role in hospital resuscitation attempts, please refer to chapter 4.

'Superfluous' personnel (if any) can be directed towards making more room around the bed/trolley area and guiding the emergency team to the collapsed patient. If relatives are present they will need support (see chapter 5), but staff should not forget that other patients on the ward or unit need care (see chapter 4).

CONCLUSION

Outcomes both in and out of hospital remain poor (see chapter 8) and in order to improve the chance of survival for the patient who has suffered a cardiorespiratory arrest, the four links of the 'Chain of Survival' (Fig. 6.2; see Checking Response, above) are essential. Out of hospital, the rescuer must:

- Ensure their own safety before approaching the victim
- Diagnose the cardiopulmonary arrest
- Call the emergency services
- Instigate and maintain BLS until the ambulance arrives.

In the hospital, the nurse must:

- Recognize the signs of deterioration and ensure that early medical intervention prevents cardiorespiratory arrest where possible.

In the event of cardiopulmonary arrest occurring, the nurse must:

- Diagnose the cardiopulmonary arrest
- Activate the emergency call system to summon the ALS team
- Instigate and maintain BLS until the ALS team arrives
- Bring the available resuscitation equipment to the patient's side
- Clear the area and prepare for ALS interventions
- Assist the resuscitation team as necessary
- Inform and support relatives and nearby patients
- Record the events accurately in the patient's nursing notes.

These measures ensure that the links of the 'Chain of Survival' are put into place.

1. Early access by recognition and alerting the emergency team.
2. Early CPR.
3. Early defibrillation.
4. Early ALS.

Resuscitation for nurses in the wards is very demanding, both professionally and personally (see chapter 4) and if they have successfully achieved points 1–4 above, they have done all they could reasonably be expected to do in ensuring patient safety. Out-of-hospital resuscitation attempts are even more difficult and, once again, if the rescuer has summoned the emergency services and instigated BLS, they too have done all that could have been done to save a life. The outcome, in both contexts, is then beyond the control of those who initiated the resuscitation attempt.

REFERENCES

American Heart Association 1992 Emergency Cardiac Care Committee and Subcommittees, American Heart Association. Guidelines for cardiopulmonary resuscitation and emergency cardiac care. Journal of American Heart Association 268:2171–2295

Bahr J, Kingler H, Panzer W, Rode H, Kettler D 1997 Skills of lay people in checking carotid pulse. Third Scientific Congress of the European Resuscitation Council (abstract). Cited in Handley et al. 1998

Baskett P, Nolan J, Parr M 1996 Tidal volumes which are perceived to be adequate for resuscitation. Resuscitation 31:231–234

Bossaert L (ed.) 1998 European Resuscitation Council guidelines for resuscitation. Elsevier, Amsterdam

Cummins R O, Ornato J P, Thies W H, Pepe P E 1991 Improving survival from sudden cardiac arrest: the 'chain of survival' concept. A statement for health professionals from the Advanced Cardiac Life Support Subcommittee and the Emergency Cardiac Care Committee, American Heart Association. Circulation 83(5):1832–1847

Eberle B, Dick W F, Schneider T, Wisser G, Doetsch S, Tzanova I 1996 Checking the carotid pulse check: diagnostic accuracy of first responders in patients with or without pulse. Resuscitation 33:107–116

European Resuscitation Council 1992 Basic Life Support Working Party of the European Resuscitation Council. Guidelines for basic life support. Resuscitation 24:103–110

Flesche C W, Brewer S, Mandel L P, Brevik H, Tarnow J 1994 The ability of health professionals to check the carotid pulse. Circulation 90(suppl 1):288

Handley A J, Becker L B, Allen M, van Drenth A, Kramer E B, Montgomery W H 1997 Single rescuer adult basic life support. An advisory statement from the basic life support working group of the international liaison committee on resuscitation (ILCOR). Resuscitation 34(2):101–108

Handley A J, Bahr J, Baskett P et al. 1998 The 1998 European Resuscitation Council guidelines for adult single rescuer basic life support. A statement from the working group on basic life support, and approved by the executive committee of the European Resuscitation Council. Resuscitation 37:67–80

Mather C, O'Kelly S 1996 The palpation of pulses. Anaesthesia 51:189–191

Resuscitation Council (UK) 1998 Advanced life support course provider manual, 3rd edn. Resuscitation Council (UK), London

UKCC 1992 Code of professional conduct, 3rd edn. UK Central Council for Nursing, Midwifery and Health Visiting, London

Advanced life support

Di Smith

INTRODUCTION

In 1992, the European Resuscitation Council (ERC) published the guidelines for advanced life support (ALS). This was a landmark in international co-operation and co-ordination (European Resuscitation Council 1992), as prior to this, different institutions and specialist societies had published various clinical guidelines. The result was that nurses and doctors were presented with difficulties when attending patients who had suffered a cardiac arrest. The difficulties resulted from an absence of uniformity and any systematic approach to resuscitation: different attending medics would use different guidelines. While it was recognized that the guidelines were there to guide the user and that variation from the guidelines may be required in different circumstances, anecdotal evidence often reflected confusion in the management of cardiac arrest.

The publication of the UK guidelines in 1989, which were then revised in 1992 (European Resuscitation Council Working Party 1993), made the management of cardiac arrest more systematic for all those involved in administering ALS. There still remained the problem of teaching the guidelines since three sets of algorithms did mean more for users to remember. The International Liaison Committee on Resuscitation (ILCOR) identified this when they published a series of advisory statements in 1997. The Resuscitation Council adopted the statements for the UK, with some minor modifications, as new guidelines for use in 1997 with the agreement to assess them on behalf of the European Resuscitation Council (Bruce-Jones 1997).

Since nurses are often involved in assisting and in some cases managing the process of ALS, this chapter sets out to clarify the use of the algorithms in ALS. The new guidelines will be given in detail, with the support of anecdotal evidence of their use in clinical practice. The anecdotal evidence is not research-based but is used to demonstrate the way that the guidelines have been applied in practice. The guidelines are just those, guidelines. In the everyday practice of nursing and medicine, the limitations of guidelines must be recognized: 'Words and flow charts must be interpreted with common sense and appreciation of their intent' (Bossaert 1998, p. 36).

The ALS Working Group for ILCOR (Chamberlain & Cummins 1997) recognized that the guidelines of 1992 required the users to be able to assess and interpret the rhythm. There would then be a requirement for decision-making which some users found difficult. The development and increasing use of automated external defibrillators (AEDs) helped to reduce the problem of rhythm recognition; however, the 1992 guidelines were not specifically designed for these devices. The new guidelines are applicable to manual and automated external defibrillators and, as a result, they are aimed at keeping decision-making to a minimum wherever possible (Bossaert 1998).

THE UNIVERSAL ALGORITHM

The changes in the universal algorithm have been made in an effort to simplify it for the user. The 1992 guidelines identified three rhythms that caused cardiac arrest, each rhythm having its own flow-chart for management.

The ALS Working Group for ILCOR (Chamberlain & Cummins 1997) recommended that a 'two arrest rhythm' approach be used. The rationale for this change was based on the recognition that there was limited scientific information, owing to the lack of available convincing human data on some aspects of resuscitation (Kloeck et al. 1997). The modifications were suggested on educational rather than scientific grounds (Kloeck et al. 1997).

The three cardinal cardiac arrest rhythms of ventricular fibrillation (VF)/pulseless ventricular tachycardia (VT), asystole and electrical mechanical dissociation (EMD) have been divided into two subsets: VF/pulseless VT and non-VF/pulseless VT (Fig. 7.1). Non-VF/pulseless VT incorporates both asystole and EMD.

Each step that follows in the ALS algorithm assumes that the preceding one has been unsuccessful (Bossaert 1998). Following an initial assessment and instigation of the universal algorithm, the rescuers are specifically directed to seek and treat the reversible causes of the cardiac arrest (Kloeck et al. 1997).

Cardiac arrest

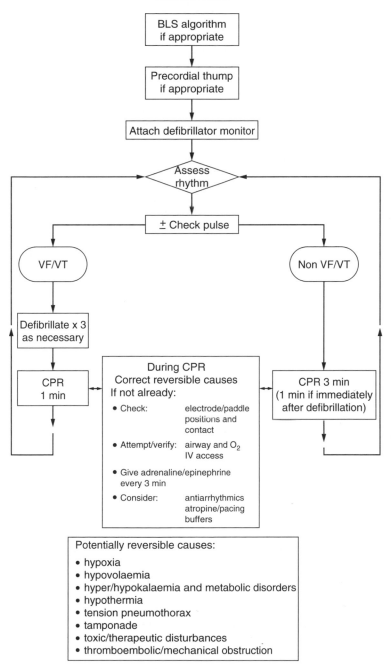

Fig. 7.1 The universal algorithm. Resuscitation Council (UK) 1998, reproduced with permission.

INITIATING THE ALS GUIDELINES

The most important first step in managing any cardiac arrest is its recognition and the commencement of basic life support (BLS) protocols. It is not the intention of the author to repeat the BLS protocols given in chapter 6; therefore, it is recommended that readers familiarize themselves with these protocols before continuing with this chapter.

In certain wards or units, patients may develop life-threatening cardiac rhythms that are not witnessed, or there is a lack of appropriately trained personnel. In this situation, it is recommended that BLS protocols be commenced.

Where the event is witnessed, a precordial thump may be sufficient to reverse a VF/VT arrhythmia to a rhythm that gives an output (Cadwell *et al.* 1985, Robertson 1992). I have known VF and pulseless VT to be reverted to a rhythm that produces an output when a precordial thump has been delivered within the first 30 s following its onset. On some occasions, the patients were still conscious and aware of their surroundings but reported afterwards that they had experienced a sense of 'impending doom'. On recognition of the event and the delivery of the precordial thump, there was no time to give extensive explanations, the patients were told that their heart had developed a problem with the rhythm and that the thump was to revert it to 'normal'. Once the emergency was over a more detailed explanation and reassurance was given. A call to the emergency team (crash call) was still made, since in previous situations patients tended to revert to VF or VT within a few minutes of the precordial thump. There were occasions, however, when senior house officers were present at the time and anti-arrhythmia drugs administered to prevent reoccurring VT/VF.

The case for the precordial thump has been put forward by Robertson (1992). In a witnessed arrest, it is a procedure identified as a class 1 recommendation in the ALS guidelines. A class 1 recommendation is defined as a definitely helpful procedure (Chamberlain & Cummins 1997). A precordial thump, if used, should precede (albeit by only a few seconds) the attachment of a monitor/defibrillator. Electrocardiogram (ECG) monitoring then provides the link between BLS and ALS procedures. ECG rhythm assessment must always be interpreted within the clinical context since movement artefact, lead disconnection and electrical interference can mimic rhythms associated with cardiac arrest (see Case history 7.1). It should also be noted that in the event where a unit/ward cardiac monitor is detached in favour of a defibrillator monitor, then the unit/ward cardiac monitor should be switched off. A colleague recalls attending a resuscitation attempt where the ward cardiac monitor was left on and the attending team was looking at this monitor instead of the defibrillating monitor, which had been attached when defibrillation began. Fortunately, this was identified quickly, so there were no detrimental consequences. Unfortunately, errors like this can easily occur in stressful circumstances.

Following the assessment of the patient for the causative arrhythmia, the algorithm splits into two pathways: VF/VT and other rhythms.

Case history 7.1

In a coronary care unit a patient being monitored appeared to be in VF. The patient was actually out of view and the response was rapid in order to act upon what appeared to be a life-threatening arrhythmia. On reaching the patient, it was clear that the diagnosis was in error, as the patient was reading a newspaper. The artefact resulted from the patient's movement and electrical interference from an infusion pump that was plugged into the electrical socket next to where the cardiac monitor socket was located.

Other, similar, events have been recounted by nurses working with cardiac patients; for example, one colleague recalled when a patient was asleep but appeared (according to the reading on the cardiac monitor) to be in asystole. However, on investigation, it was found that one of the cardiac monitor leads had become unattached.

These accounts may appear humorous, but they are stressful for both the nurse and patient concerned. The important point is to check the patient first for a response (see chapter 6).

VF/VT RHYTHMS

In adults, the most common primary arrhythmia at the onset of cardiac arrest is VF or pulseless VT (Adgey *et al.* 1982, Deluna *et al.* 1989, Sedgewick *et al.* 1994). There is evidence that states that the majority of survivors come from this group (Roth *et al.* 1984, Tortolani *et al.* 1990, Tunstall-Pedoe *et al.* 1992, Ekstrom *et al.* 1994). If the definitive therapy for this arrhythmia – defibrillation – can be implemented promptly, a perfusing cardiac rhythm may be restored and lead to ultimate survival. The only interventions that have been shown to improve long-term survival are BLS and early defibrillation (Robertson *et al.* 1998). On identifying VF/pulseless VT as the causative rhythm, then the left-hand side of the algorithm should be followed (Fig. 7.2).

In out-of-hospital cardiac arrest, and in most hospital settings, BLS will usually have been initiated before the algorithm for ventricular fibrillation or pulseless ventricular tachycardia is commenced. If the cardiac arrest occurs in the hospital setting and immediate defibrillation is possible – for example in a high-dependency area where a rapidly charging defibrillator is available – a precordial thump should be given before the definitive electrical treatment (Chamberlain *et al.* 1992).

VF is a notably treatable rhythm, but the chances of successful defibrillation decline subsequently with the passage of each minute (Neumar *et al.* 1990, Cobbe *et al.* 1991). The amplitude and waveform of VF deteriorate rapidly, reflecting the depletion of myocardial high-energy phosphate stores (Mapin *et al.* 1991). The rate of decline in success depends, in part, upon the provision and adequacy of BLS (Larsen *et al.* 1993), but early defibrillation

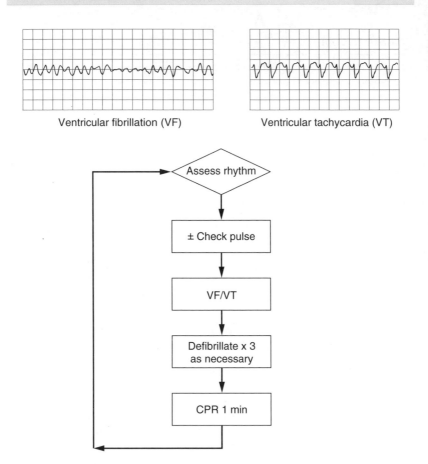

Ventricular fibrillation (VF)   Ventricular tachycardia (VT)

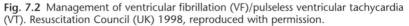

Fig. 7.2 Management of ventricular fibrillation (VF)/pulseless ventricular tachycardia (VT). Resuscitation Council (UK) 1998, reproduced with permission.

is a more significant contributor to a positive outcome. Therefore, the priority is to minimize any delay between the onset of cardiac arrest and the administration of defibrillating shocks. The delivery of a group of three shocks (the initial sequence should have energies of 200 J, 200 J and 360 J) was retained in the ALS guidelines of 1997 (Robertson *et al.* 1998; see chapter 10 for details on defibrillation).

PRESERVATION OF CEREBRAL FUNCTION

Over 80% of individuals successfully defibrillated will have this achieved by one of the first three shocks (Hargenten *et al.* 1990, Cobbe *et al.* 1991, Tunstall-Pedoe *et al.* 1992). If the first three shocks have been unsuccessful, the outlook for recovery is poor, but not hopeless; attempts should therefore continue if this strategy is appropriate on clinical grounds, for example in young myocardial infarct victims. If this happens, then delay in restoration of a coordinated rhythm is inevitable. Subsequently, the best prospects for restoring a perfusing rhythm will remain with defibrillation (see chapter 10), but at this stage the search for and correction of potentially reversible causes or aggravating factors is indicated (Robertson *et al*. 1998).

The priority then changes to preservation of cerebral function by the best possible BLS, while delaying as far as possible further myocardial deterioration (Chamberlain *et al*. 1992). BLS is commenced for 1 min, which is approximately 10 cycles of five compressions to one ventilation breath. During this time, efforts are made to secure the airway using advanced airway techniques and to access the circulatory system for the delivery of drugs (Robertson *et al*. 1998).

ADVANCED AIRWAY MANAGEMENT

A brief attempt should be made at this time to intubate the patient. Tracheal intubation remains the optimal procedure (Robertson *et al*. 1998). It is recognized that this procedure can sometimes be hazardous and it requires a skilled operator to complete the manoeuvre successfully. The laryngeal mask airway offers an alternative to tracheal intubation. It is a relatively easy technique to learn and many hospital trusts have invested in training nursing personnel in carrying out this procedure. It should be noted, however, that it does not guarantee absolutely against aspiration (Brimacombe & Berry 1995, Owens *et al*. 1995; see chapter 9). Whichever technique is used, the ultimate aim is to deliver the highest possible concentration of oxygen into the patient's lungs, preferably 100% (Resuscitation Council (UK) 1998).

In the event that a skilled rescuer is not available to intubate using either of the above techniques, then it is recommended that the airway be maintained using the bag-valve mask unit as a two-person technique (Resuscitation Council (UK) 1998).

DRUG DELIVERY

If intravenous (IV) access is not already available, it must be acquired. The peripheral venous route remains the optimal method of drug administration during cardiopulmonary resuscitation (Robertson *et al*. 1998). If intravenous access is not in place at the time of cardiac arrest, then a cannula with a relatively large diameter of 1.2 mm or 1.4 mm sited in the antecubital vein is recommended in adults (Hapnes & Robertson 1992). More distal veins should be avoided because of the longer time needed for the drugs to reach the central circulation (i.e. great vessels and heart).

Since more and more qualified nurses are adding venous cannulation to their repertoire, this is an aspect of ALS that can be accomplished by nursing staff, if BLS is being performed.

Where peripheral venous cannulation and drug delivery is used, a flush of 20 mL of 0.9% saline is advised in order to expedite entry of the drugs to the circulation (Resuscitation Council (UK) 1998). A technique referred to as 'milking' the limb, which involves raising the limb in which the drug is being delivered and stroking it in a downwards motion towards the body in order to speed up the delivery of the drug to the central circulation, may also be used.

When nursing staff are involved in participating in a resuscitation attempt, managing the delivery of drugs can present a challenge. Many trusts have invested in pre drawn up emergency drugs. These drugs are simple to prepare for administration. They are supplied in a box that is clearly labelled and has the drug already in the vial of the syringe barrel, which is prevented from leaking by a rubber bung. An injector is also supplied in the box. Both the injector and the syringe have a cap which is removed when the drug is required and the injector is inserted into the syringe barrel. The injector has a metal prong within it that will pierce the rubber bung in the barrel if the injector is inserted and then twisted clockwise three times. This method of drug delivery reduces the risk of needle stick injury since it removes the task of drawing up drug from a drug vial using a separate needle and syringe. It is advised, however, that personnel involved in preparing and using these drugs should have training. One problem has been reported, anecdotally, with pre drawn up drugs. One of the doctors participating in a resuscitation attempt was handed a pre drawn up syringe of adrenaline (epinephrine). However, the drug ampoule was not fully wound into the barrel of the syringe, which resulted in the doctor having trouble in delivering the drug into the cannula. To reduce the risk of this happening, users are advised to thread the vial into the injector and twist the vial three and a half turns clockwise until the needle penetrates the vial stopper and comes into contact with the medication.

It should also be noted that, to avoid errors, when assisting with this aspect of resuscitation the nurse should check the drug to be administered with the doctor who is to give the drug. Nurses are not legally covered to give emergency drugs without prescription; the responsibility lies with the doctor to check the drug before giving it.

There is some debate about the position of the nurse when administering adrenaline in the event of the drug not being prescribed. Clause one of the *Code of Professional Conduct* states that 'the nurse must always act in such a manner as to promote and safeguard the interests and well-being of patients and client' (UKCC 1992a). It could therefore be argued that in the event of a cardiac arrest, the nurse who has kept up to date and is able to recognize that adrenaline is required, should administer it. The nurse would then ensure that it is reported to the attending resuscitation team and recorded on the patient' notes/drug charts. However, the UKCC (1992b) *Standards for the Administration of Medicines* (clause 6.12) clearly states that 'where it is the wish of the professional staff concerned that practitioners (nurses) in a particular setting be authorized to administer, on their own authority, certain medicines, a local protocol has been agreed between medical practitioners, nurses and midwives and the pharmacist'. The nurse is not legally covered to administer drugs that have not been prescribed unless a protocol has been agreed.

If pre drawn up drugs are not used, then the alternative is to draw up the drugs from ampoules using a separate needle and syringe. This can be hazardous as errors and injury can occur in the heat of the moment. Injury can be minimized by the person drawing up the drugs keeping their elbows tucked into their sides to reduce shaking.

If a central line is already *in situ*, then this route is preferred since drug delivery to the central circulation will be rapid (Robertson *et al.* 1998).

None of the above procedures should be allowed to cause undue delay in the continuation of either BLS or administration of further shocks. The person leading the resuscitation procedure should allow a limited time, perhaps 15 s, before chest compression and ventilation are continued, (Chamberlain *et al.* 1992).

There have been trials of new techniques, most notably with active compression–decompression (ACD) CPR. However, these trials are ongoing and currently there are no clinical data to show unequivocal improvement in outcomes (Nolan *et al.* 1998).

THE USE OF ADRENALINE

Adrenaline, also known as epinephrine, which has been adopted by ILCOR, has been the adrenergic amine favoured for the management of human cardiac arrest for almost 30 years (Tang *et al.* 1991). Experimentally, adrenaline has been shown to improve myocardial, cerebral blood flow and resuscitation rates in animals (Redding & Pearson 1963a). It has also been reported that doses higher than the standard dose of 1 mg are more effective (Redding & Pearson 1963b). However, studies by Woodhouse *et al.* (1995) and Herlitz *et al.* (1995a) reported that there was no clinical evidence for adrenaline improving survival or neurological recovery in humans, regardless of whether a standard or high dose of adrenaline is used. There have been some clinical trials that have reported slightly increased rates of spontaneous circulation with the use of high-dose adrenaline (Steill *et al.* 1992, Abramson *et al.* 1995); however, these studies showed that there was no improvement in the overall survival rate. To add to the debate, studies by Tang *et al.* (1991) report pulmonary/ventilation defects induced by adrenaline during cardiopulmonary resuscitation. Tang *et al.* (1995) also reported that the higher dose of adrenaline increases the severity of post-resuscitation myocardial dysfunction. Both studies apply to animals and there is a lack of human trials to support these findings. In the absence of research evidence to the contrary, adrenaline 1 mg should be given via the IV route every 3 min in adults (Resuscitation Council (UK) 1998).

In practice, monitoring the time factor is not always practical. Given that the process of rhythm assessment, delivery of three DC shocks and 1 min of CPR takes 2–3 min, some practitioners have given adrenaline with each loop of the algorithm. Robertson *et al.* (1998) support this practice. In some Trusts, the resuscitation training officers have introduced stop clocks to the resuscitation trolleys. In the event of a cardiac arrest, the staff simply hit the on button when the first dose of adrenaline is administered. The clock is set to alarm every 3 min, thus reminding the team that the next dose of adrenaline is to be given (if required).

The role of adrenaline is to improve the efficacy of BLS; it is not an adjunct to defibrillation (Chamberlain *et al.* 1992). The α-adrenergic effect causes arteriolar vasoconstriction thus diverting blood away from nonessential organs.

Adrenaline will normally be administered before the next set of defibrillating shocks, but it is recommended that the delivery of shocks should not be delayed for drug treatment (Chamberlain *et al.* 1992). The interval between the third and fourth shocks should not exceed 2 min and although the interventions that can be performed during this period may improve the prospects of successful defibrillation, this is not proven. However, it is well established that with the passage of time, the chance of success for defibrillating shocks lessens (Robertson *et al.* 1998).

IDENTIFICATION AND CORRECTION OF REVERSIBLE CAUSES

For the patient with persistent VF/VT, potential causes or aggravating factors may include electrolyte imbalance, hypothermia and drug or toxic agents for which specific treatment may be indicated. It is an important role of the nurse, therefore, to make the attending medics (who may not know the patient) aware what the patient's condition was prior to the arrest and what medication the patient was/is on.

Electrolyte abnormalities that cause cardiac arrest are uncommon, except in the case of hyperkalaemia (ILCOR 1997; for identification and treatment of hyperkalaemia, see under causes of EMD below).

LOOPING THE ALGORITHM

Following 1 min of BLS while the various interventions have been explored and/or initiated, the next series of three shocks are given at 360 J. This is then followed by another minute of BLS, giving time to secure advanced airway and ventilation techniques, oxygenation and drug delivery (if not already achieved). At this stage, anti-arrhythmic drugs may be considered.

ANTI-ARRHYTHMIC DRUGS

Anti-arrhythmic drugs may be considered following the first two sets of three shocks. It is acceptable to maintain the previous policy of deferring this treatment until after four sets of shocks have been given (Robertson *et al.* 1998).

Lignocaine

Lignocaine, also known as lidocaine (Bruce-Jones 1997), appears to remain the drug of choice in managing arrhythmias. Despite various studies, some of which report that lignocaine increases the defibrillating threshold in animals (Dorain *et al.* 1986, Natale *et al.* 1991), a study by Lake *et al.* (1986) using a randomized placebo-controlled trial, reported beneficial effects on the threshold of patients undergoing myocardial reperfusion after coronary artery bypass. Until the results of further trials are published, it is recommended that no change be made to the use of lignocaine, bretylium and other anti-arrhythmic agents (Robertson *et al.* 1998).

Lignocaine is used for the treatment of refractory VF and haemodynamically stable VT. An initial rapid IV dose (over 2 min) of either 100 mg for VF or 1 mg/kg for haemodynamically stable VT is recommended (Resuscitation Council (UK) 1998). This initial dose is rapidly distributed throughout the body and is effective for only 20 min. This may be repeated once and followed, if required, by an infusion of 2–4 mg/min to achieve a constant therapeutic effect (Resuscitation Council (UK) 1998). Lignocaine acts by suppressing the excitability of the ventricular muscle with only moderate depression of heart action (Trounce 1994), thereby reducing the incidence of primary VF after acute myocardial infarction. During cardiac arrest normal clearance mechanisms do not function, thus high plasma concentrations may be achieved after a single dose. Lignocaine toxicity produces paraesthesia, drowsiness, confusion and muscular twitching progressing to convulsions. Lignocaine is less effective in the presence of hypokalaemia and hypomagnesaemia.

Bretylium tosylate

Bretylium tosylate is used for the treatment of refractory VT and VF. It is an adrenergic neurone-blocking agent. Blockade with inhibition of further release of noradrenaline (norepinephrine) starts about 20 min after injection. The drug also inhibits uptake into nerve terminals, which may potentiate the effects of adrenaline administered. The duration of both the action potential and the effective refractory period is increased in normal muscle and Purkinje tissue.

The effects of bretylium are poorly understood and although it raises the threshold for VF there is debate about its effect on the defibrillation threshold. The anti-arrhythmic effects may take some time to become established. Therefore, BLS must be continued for at least 20 min after administration. The nurse should continue monitoring the patient's vital signs as hypotension may follow successful conversion of VF and require plasma volume expansion (Resuscitation Council (UK) 1998).

USE OF BUFFER AGENTS

Arterial blood gas analysis does not show a rapid or severe development of acidosis during cardiopulmonary arrest if effective BLS is carried out (Steedman & Robertson 1992). Acidaemia may be measured by analysis of arterial or mixed venous samples. The results may be misleading, however, and bear little relation to the actual internal milieu of cerebral or myocardial intracellular values (Caparelli *et al.* 1989, Kette *et al.* 1993). For this reason, the role of buffers in CPR remains uncertain. It is suggested that the judicial use of buffers be limited only to severe acidosis (arterial pH < 7.1 and base excess > −10) (Robertson *et al.* 1998). The amount of sodium bicarbonate required can be calculated using the following formula:

Base excess × body weight (kg)/3

(Advanced Life Support Group 1993, p. 35)

Further administration will depend upon fresh blood gas analysis and the clinical situation (Robertson *et al.* 1998). In situations where blood gas analysis is not possible, the Resuscitation Council (UK) (1998) asserts that it is reasonable to consider sodium bicarbonate after 20–25 min, particularly if the resuscitation was delayed or suboptimal. A dose of 50 mmol (50 mL of an 8.4% solution) is recommended.

Caution should be taken if administered with calcium as the solution is incompatible with calcium salts, causing precipitation with calcium carbonate (Resuscitation Council (UK) 1998).

NON-VF/VT

The survival rates for patients with these rhythms are much less favourable than for those with VF/VT (Herlitz *et al.* 1995b), unless a reversible cause

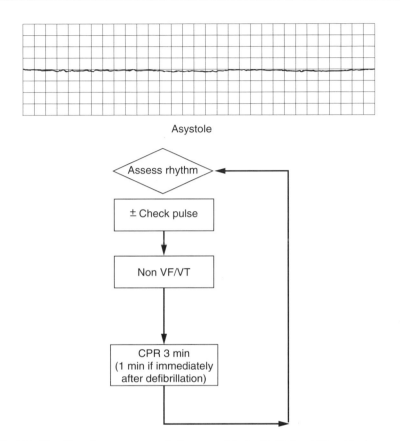

Asystole

Assess rhythm

± Check pulse

Non VF/VT

CPR 3 min
(1 min if immediately
after defibrillation)

Fig. 7.3 Algorithm for management of non-ventricular fibrillation VF/ventricular tachycardia (VT). Resuscitation Council (UK) 1998, reproduced with permission.

can be found and effectively treated (Resuscitation Council (UK) 1998). If VF/VT were positively excluded, defibrillation would not be used as a primary intervention. In this instance, the right-sided path of the algorithm is followed (Fig. 7.3).

ASYSTOLE

Asystole carries a poorer prognosis than VF or pulseless VT. It must be recognized that asystole may appear on the cardiac monitor, when in fact it is fine VF. It is essential that the correct diagnosis be made since VF is a treatable rhythm. The leads should be checked and the gain setting on the monitor increased to exclude VF. If there is any doubt then treatment should begin as if for VF. Note that 'The risks of not treating VF, with its greater potential for a successful outcome, are greater than applying three (unnecessary) shocks' (Resuscitation Council (UK) 1998, p. 59).

BLS should be performed for 3 min. During BLS advanced airway management and ventilation techniques should be performed, venous access secured and the first dose of adrenaline 1 mg given.

Atropine 3 mg is given IV; 6 mg may be given by the endotracheal route, but in no greater volume than 20 mL (Resuscitation Council (UK) 1998). The action of atropine is to antagonize the parasympathetic neurotransmitter acetylcholine at muscarinic receptors; i.e. the inherent features that the sinoatrial (SA) node has to initiate electrical impulses are no longer slowed by the action of the vagus nerve. The result of blocking the effect of acetylcholine released by the vagus nerve will allow the SA node to fire its impulses more rapidly. Electrical stimulation from the SA node then increases the rate of electrical impulses from the atrioventricular (AV) node, resulting in an increase in heart rate and cardiac output. This is a once-only dose as atropine has half-life of 4 h (Hardman 1996). Side-effects of atropine include dry mouth, urinary urgency and retention, flushing and dryness of the skin, dilation of the pupils and loss of accommodation, photophobia and occasionally confusion (particularly in the elderly) (British Medical Association & Royal Pharmaceutical Society of Great Britain 1999).

Where the diagnosis of asystole is made, the ECG should be carefully checked for the presence of 'p' waves or slow ventricular activity. These arrhythmias may respond to cardiac pacing, which may be external or transvenous, depending on the equipment available and the skills of the attending resuscitation team members (Resuscitation Council (UK) 1998).

Dowdle (1996) reported a technique referred to as external cardiac percussion. This technique involves the delivery of a series of gentle blows over the precordium, using the heel of the hand and delivering lighter blows than that for a precordial thump. The result was the generation of a succession of virtually unbroken QRS complexes. The patient, who had a pacemaker *in situ* that had failed to capture, had his cardiac output maintained for 15 min while X-ray screening was being set up and the pacing wire adjusted. In the same paper, Dowdle recounted an incident described by D. Chamberlain (personal communication) of how a patient in ventricular standstill was transferred by ambulance with the accompanying paramedic carrying out cardiac percussion. This maintained the patient near normal cardiac output levels throughout the transfer. Robertson *et al.* (1998) report that the rate at which external cardiac percussion is performed is the same as the rate for external cardiac massage (100/min).

If, during resuscitation of patients in asystole, the rhythm changes to VF, then the left side of the algorithm is followed (see Figs 7.1 and 7.2). If asystole continues then BLS continues while reversible or aggravating factors are identified and treated. Adrenaline is administered every 3 min but if after three loops there has been no response then high-dose adrenaline (5 mg) may be considered as a once-only dose (Resuscitation Council (UK) 1998). Robertson *et al.* (1998) advise that resuscitation attempts for asystolic patients should generally continue for at least 20–30 min from the time of collapse, unless there are overwhelming reasons to believe that resuscitation is hopeless.

ELECTROMECHANICAL DISSOCIATION (EMD)

This condition, also known as pulseless electrical activity (PEA), gives the clinical signs of cardiac arrest, but an ECG rhythm, which would normally be associated with a cardiac output. The best chance of survival in this instance is prompt assessment to find and treat the cause. While this is being done, resuscitation must continue, following the right side of the universal algorithm (Fig. 7.3). BLS is commenced immediately and advanced airway management and ventilation performed as required. Access to the circulation should be gained and adrenaline 1 mg IV given every 3 min.

Causes of EMD

Potentially reversible causes have been identified and divided into two groups of four based on their initial letter (either H or T). This is to aid the memory of those managing cardiac arrests (Resuscitation Council (UK) 1998).

Hypoxia

Hypoxia can be described to as a reduction in tissue oxygenation. Common causes are airway obstruction, which may or may not be associated with chronic obstructive pulmonary disease (COPD), heart failure, and/or circulatory shock. Acute respiratory failure associated with asthma is an increasingly common cause. Intubating the patient with a cuffed endotracheal tube and ventilating with 100% oxygen eliminates hypoxia best. If it is not possible to achieve this, then one of the airway procedures outlined above or in chapter 9 should be attempted.

Hypovolaemia

Hypovolaemia in adults that results in EMD may occur because of blood loss. Trauma is an obvious cause. Other factors that the nurse needs to consider are:

- Does the patient have a history of gastric bleeding; are there any signs such as haematemesis and malaena?
- Is the patient receiving thrombolytic therapy?
- Has a diagnosis, provisional or otherwise, been made of aortic aneurysm?

While it is not the nurse's role to make a medical diagnosis, they may be aware of significant factors in the history of the patient who has developed EMD. The key intervention for hypovolaemia is identifying and stopping the source of fluid loss and administration of fluid to replace circulating volume (Thelan *et al.* 1994). The type of fluids administered may be in the form of crystalloid or colloid, or a combination of both.

Crystalloids and colloids

Crystalloids are balanced electrolyte solutions. Examples of these solutions are sodium chloride, lactated Ringer's solution and dextrose 5% in water (Thelan *et al.* 1994). Colloids are protein- or starch-containing solutions such as blood or blood components. Other types of colloid solutions are pharmaceutical plasma expanders such as Manitol, Dextran 70 and Hexastarch. The choice of solution will depend on the situation (Thelan *et al.* 1994). If haemorrhage is the cause of the hypovolaemic shock then the use of colloids has the advantage of rapidly restoring the intravascular volume with a smaller amount of fluids. The disadvantages are allergic reactions. Difficulty may occur with cross-matching the patient for further blood, therefore a sample of blood will be required prior to the administration of colloids (British Medical Association & Royal Pharmaceutical Society of Great Britain 1999). While resuscitation is continued, urgent arrangements are made to transfer the patient to the operating theatre for surgery to stop the bleeding.

Hyperkalaemia, hypokalaemia and other metabolic disorders

These disorders may only become known when biochemistry results are received. If it is known that the patient has a metabolic disorder or is on medication such as calcium channel blockers then these factors need to be communicated to the attending medics.

Hyperkalaemia is a condition where there is an increase in serum potassium above 5.0 mEq/L in the blood (Bear & Myers 1994). Patients who are hyperkalaemic and are being monitored, may have shown tenting of the T waves prior to the arrest (Fig. 7.4). Hyperkalaemia is more dangerous than hypokalaemia (low serum potassium) because it has a profound effect on myocardial muscle, which may result in cardiac arrest (Bear & Myers 1994). The patients who are most at risk are those with renal failure or Addison's disease. Nursing staff should also be aware of the potential problems of hyperkalaemia associated with patients receiving too rapid an IV infusion containing potassium. The choice of drug regimen will depend upon the severity of the hyperkalaemia.

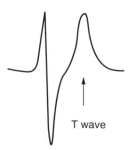

T wave

Fig. 7.4 Tenting of T waves in hyperkalaemia.

Table 7.1 Common causes of cardiac instability caused by electrolyte imbalance

Electrolyte	Common causes	ECG changes	Treatment
Hypokalaemia (less than 3.5 mEq/L K⁺)	Diuretics Excessive vomiting and/or diarrhoea Respiratory or metabolic acidosis Gastric suction Post insulin administration	Slightly peaked T wave Slightly prolonged P–R interval Shallow, wide, flat or inverted T wave Prominent U wave	Potassium replacement Magnesium
Hyperkalaemia (greater than 5.5 mEq/L K⁺)	Renal failure Endocrine disorders – Addison's disease	Tenting T waves (see Fig. 7.4) Prolonged P–R interval, Smaller P waves, QRS widening (McCance & Huether 1994) VT, VF, asystole	Calcium chloride Bicarbonate IV insulin and glucose IV or inhaled beta agonist Dialysis (ILCOR 1997)
Hypomagnesaemia (less than 1.5 mEq/L Mg²⁺)	Malnutrition associated with alcoholism Urinary loss GI loss Malabsorption	Prolongation of QT conduction Shortened ST segment Broad T waves Ventricular tachycardia Ventricular fibrillation Asystole Bradycardia	Magnesium sulphate
Hypomagnesaemia (greater than 2.5 mEq/L Mg²⁺)	Rare, usually associated with renal failure Magnesium-containing antacids can potentiate excess magnesium	Atrioventricular block Asystole	Calcium chloride (ILCOR 1997) Dialysis
Hypocalcaemia (less than 8.5 mg/dL Ca²⁺)	Hypothyroidism Acute pancreatitis Renal failure	Prolongation of QT conduction Elevated ST segment Peaked or inverted T waves	Calcium chloride (ILCOR 1997)

In EMD where hyperkalaemia is the cause, then 10 mL of 10% (6.8 Ca^{2+}) calcium chloride may be given as an initial dose and repeated if necessary (Resuscitation Council (UK) 1998). Calcium acts quickly to protect the myocardium by antagonizing the effect of hyperkalaemia on the heart (Trounce 1994). However, calcium may have detrimental effects on the ischaemic myocardium and may impair cerebral recovery. It is given in an arrest situation only if there are specific indications for its use (Resuscitation Council (UK) 1998). If the patient is receiving digitalis therapy the nurse needs to be aware that calcium administration sensitizes the heart to digitalis, which may result in digitalis intoxication (Bear & Myers 1994). Common electrolyte imbalances that are causes of cardiac arrest are given in Table 7.1.

Hypothermia

Hypothermia is often associated with drowning or near drowning. It is also associated with elderly patients who have an underactive thyroid gland. Hypothermia is defined as a patient who has a core temperature of below 35 °C (Advanced Life Support Group 1993). Hypothermia increases the tolerance time for cardiac arrest, thus making the case for prolonged resuscitation attempts. This author has often heard the phrase that 'a patient can be warm and dead but not cold and dead'. It is not therefore surprising that warming the patient while maintaining BLS becomes a priority, but one that cannot be rushed. The removal of wet clothes and the application of dry blankets should prevent further heat loss. Patients can be rewarmed by internal active rewarming, such as the introduction of warmed intravenous saline 0.9% at 42–46 °C, oesophageal rewarming tubes or peritoneal lavage at 42–44 °C (Resuscitation Council (UK) 1998). Successful resuscitation without neurological deficit has been reported after 70 min of cardiac arrest followed by 2 h of BLS before active rewarming was started by cardiopulmonary bypass (ILCOR 1997).

Hypothermia results in a reduced blood flow during resuscitation, possibly owing to lowered metabolic rate and inhibition of deleterious effects of hypoxia such as free radical reactions and changes in cell membrane permeability. Severe hypothermia can cause bradycardia. As a result, the heart may have a reduced response to pacemaker stimulation, defibrillation and drugs. Drugs may also accumulate to toxic levels. If the core temperature is < 30 °C, then ILCOR (1997) recommends a maximum of three shocks for VF/VT until the core temperature is increased.

Tension pneumothorax

Tension pneumothorax usually results from injury that causes perforation to the chest wall or pleura (Thelan *et al.* 1994). It occurs when the opening into the pleural space from the lung or the outside chest wall acts as a one-way valve allowing air to enter that space during inhalation. During exhalation, air is trapped in the pleural space (Alexander *et al.* 1994), resulting in a build-up of air in the pleural space on the affected side causing an increase in pressure leading to mediastinal shift to the opposite side. Pressure continues to build, resulting in pressure on the heart and thoracic aorta. This leads to a decrease in venous return and decreased cardiac output (Thelan *et al*. 1994). Tension pneumothorax may be the primary cause of EMD or it may occur following insertion of a catheter into a central vein (Rutter 1995). The diagnosis is made by clinical assessment since there is no time for chest X-ray as this life-threatening condition needs immediate attention. The signs are: development of difficulty in breathing, increased respiratory rate and pulse with laboured breathing and unequal chest expansion. The patient may also experience sudden chest pain extending to the shoulders. The neck veins become distended and the patient may become cyanosed (Thelan *et al*. 1994). If pulse oximetry is used, the oxygen saturation will drop and the blood pressure will fall. Clinical examination will yield absent breath sounds on the affected side and tracheal deviation may be observed as the trachea shifts away from the injured side. Percussion on the affected side reveals hyper-resonant sounds caused by the trapped air (Thelan *et al*. 1994).

On suspecting that a patient has developed a tension pneumothorax, the doctors should be notified immediately and the head of the patient's bed elevated, 100% oxygen administered (Rutter 1995) and a large-bore (14 gauge) catheter over needle should be collected, ready for insertion on arrival of the doctor. The doctor will insert the needle into the second intercostal space at the mid-clavicular line. As the needle is introduced, a loud hissing noise will be heard (Rutter 1995). As soon as it is possible, arrangements will be made to insert a chest tube and underwater seal drain.

It is unusual for bilateral tension pneumothorax to occur simultaneously, but it can occur (see Case history 7.2).

Case history 7.2

A patient suffered from chronic obstructive airways disease and received bronchodilators via nebulized air. The patient suddenly became very distressed and cyanosed. In an effort to attract attention, he stood up and appeared to be having a seizure. Collapse quickly ensued and the initial ABC assessment showed absent breathing and pulse. The emergency call was made and BLS commenced. A cardiac monitor was attached and showed electrical activity. The on-call anaesthetist was the first of the emergency team to arrive and made the diagnosis of tension pneumothorax almost immediately after her arrival.

As a temporary measure, a large-bore needle was inserted into the chest, as described above. A 20 mL syringe, plunger removed and filled with sterile water, was then attached to the needle, thus acting as an underwater seal drain. The same procedure was repeated on the other side of the chest. Spontaneous breathing had not returned so the patient's airway was secured using the endotracheal method and ventilation commenced. Arrangements were made to transfer the patient to the intensive care unit, where chest drains were set up and ready for insertion on arrival. This patient made a full recovery and returned to the ward 10 days later. He was discharged the following week.

Tamponade

Tamponade or to cardiac tamponade is described as the progressive accumulation of blood in the pericardial sac, increasing intracardial pressure and compromising the atria and ventricles (Thelan *et al.* 1994). The classic signs associated with this condition are those of Beck's triad (the presence of distended neck veins, hypotension and muffled heart sounds), which may be obscured by the arrest itself (Resuscitation Council (UK) 1998). The major nursing diagnosis for this condition is the decreased cardiac output. Treatment is aimed at relieving the tamponade by needle pericardiocentesis. This involves the aspiration of fluid from the pericardium by use of a wide-bore needle. This procedure will be carried out by the doctors once the diagnosis has been made but BLS is commenced according to the non-VF algorithm.

Thromboembolic or mechanical obstruction

Thromboembolic or mechanical obstruction is commonly caused by pulmonary embolus. Anecdotal reports of the use of vigorous cardiac compressions have been made and said to be effective. However, the definitive treatment requires facilities for cardiopulmonary bypass to allow operative removal of the clot (Resuscitation Council (UK) 1998).

Toxic or therapeutic disturbances

Cardiac arrest due to toxic disturbances is not uncommon (Table 7.2). It is important that, in order to increase the chances of survival, the basic principles of rapidly restoring circulation and ventilation apply. The next priority is the reversal of the toxin, if possible. Knowledge of the potential toxin or the recognition of clinical signs that occur can be the key to successful resuscitation (ILCOR 1997).

PERI-ARREST RHYTHMS

It is recognized that certain arrhythmias may precede or result in ventricular fibrillation (Resuscitation Council (UK) 1998). In the immediate post-arrest period, the successfully resuscitated patient is also susceptible to these arrhythmias. It is important that the nurse caring for the patient who has had, or who is at risk of having a cardiac arrest, is able to recognize the rhythm and alert the medical staff urgently. Knowledge of the peri-arrest rhythms and their protocols may reduce the incidence of cardiac arrest occurring.

The Resuscitation Council (UK) (1998) identifies three important arrhythmias that are now taught on ALS courses. These are bradycardia, broad complex tachycardia and narrow complex tachycardia. The principles of treatment are based on asking two questions. These are

1. How is the patient?
2. What is the rhythm?

The protocols have been set out to help the user to identify what actions to take when the rhythm has been identified.

Table 7.2 Drug/toxins commonly associated with cardiac instability

Drug/Toxin	Action	Effects of overdose	Management
Betablockers, e.g. propranolol, oxyprenolol, atenolol, sotalol	All betablockers slow the heart rate and may induce myocardial depression. Betablockers compete with receptor sites on the cells so that they block the effect of the naturally occurring substance	Lightheadedness Dizziness, syncope Bradycardia Hypotension Ventricular tachycardia (sotolol) Torsades de Points (British Medical Association & Royal Pharmaceutical Society of Great Britain 1999)	Atropine 3 mg as per ALS protocol If cardiogenic shock is unresponsive to atropine, IV glucagon 50–150 μg/kg in glucose 5% (British Medical Association & Royal Pharmaceutical Society of Great Britain 1999) If glucagon is not available IV isoprenaline – up to 200 μg/min or adrenaline infusion (ILCOR 1997)
Calcium channel blockers, e.g. Adalat Retard, nifedipine, nimodipine, verapamil	Interfere with the inward placement of calcium ions through slow channels of active cell membranes Myocardial contractility may be reduced, the formation and propagation of electrical impulses within the heart may be depressed Actions differ, depending on the drug	Depression of cardiac function Hypotension Complete heart block and sudden circulatory collapse has been reported (British Medical Association & Royal Pharmaceutical Society of Great Britain 1999)	Calcium chloride 10 mL 10% (6.8 mmol) repeated as required (Resuscitation Council (UK) 1998) Adrenaline infusion (ILCOR 1997) if circulatory collapse is prominent
Chloral hydrate and derivatives, e.g. Welldorm	Hypnotic and sedative actions	Cardiac arrhythmias Cardiac arrest (Reynolds 1993) Vomiting Hypotension and shock	Gastric lavage and administration of activated charcoal Symptomatic and supportive therapy with particular attention being paid to maintaining cardiovascular, respiratory and renal function (British Medical Association & Royal Pharmaceutical Society of Great Britain 1999)

Table 7.2 (contd)

Drug/Toxin	Action	Effects of overdose	Management
Cyclic antidepressants, e.g. amitriptylin, imiprimine	Prevents the uptake of amines at the nerve endings in the brain, thus increasing the concentration of amines available for receptor uptake (Trounce 1994)	Dry mouth, dilated pupils, tachycardia, cardiac depression, hypotension, cardiac arrhythmias, respiratory failure, urinary retention, visual and auditory hallucinations during recovery, metabolic acidosis	Activated charcoal by mouth or gastric lavage. Maintain airway and ventilation. IV diazepam for convulsions. Arrhythmias may respond to correction of hypoxia and acidosis. The use of antiarrhythmia drugs is best avoided (British Medical Association & Royal Pharmaceutical Society of Great Britain 1999)
Coproxamol	Analgesia	Coma, depressed respiration, pinpoint pupils. Patient may die of acute cardiovascular collapse before reaching hospital (particularly if alcohol has been consumed) (British Medical Association & Royal Pharmaceutical Society of Great Britain 1999)	Naloxone 0.8–2 mg IV repeated at intervals of 2–3 min to a maximum of 10 mg if respiratory function does not improve (British Medical Association & Royal Pharmaceutical Society of Great Britain 1999)
Cocaine	Is a local anaesthetic used for surface anaesthesia only (because of its dependence effects)	Stimulates the central nervous system causing agitation, dilated pupils, hypertension, hallucinations, hypertonia and hyperflexia. Convulsions, coma and metabolic acidosis	Sedation with IV diazepam to control convulsions. IV propranolol may be indicated for severe arrhythmias (labetalol may be preferred if there is associated hypotension) (British Medical Association & Royal Pharmaceutical Society of Great Britain 1999, p. 24)

Substance	Description	Signs/symptoms	Treatment
Cyanides	Interfere with oxygen uptake by cells by inhibition of enzymes necessary for cellular oxygen transport. Used for the eradication of rodents in industry	With large doses unconsciousness occurs within seconds and death ensues within minutes. Smaller toxic doses produce constriction of the throat, nausea, vomiting, giddiness, headache, palpitations, hyperpnoea then dyspnoea, tachycardia followed by bradycardia. Unconsciousness followed by convulsions. Smell of bitter almonds	Dicobalt edetate is one antidote, but it is toxic and is recommended to be used only if the patient is losing or has lost consciousness. IV 300 mg (20 mL over 1–5 min if the condition is less serious) (British Medical Association & Royal Pharmaceutical Society of Great Britain 1999). Sodium nitrate. Sodium thiosulphate
Digoxin	A cardiac glycoside that has positive inotropic effects (increases contractility of the heart muscle) and negative chronotropic effects (reduces heart rate). Increases vagal tone. Decreases sympathetic drive. Prolongs atrioventricular conduction	Almost any cardiac arrhythmia. Anorexia, nausea, vomiting, diarrhoea, abdominal pain, visual disturbances, drowsiness, confusion, delirium, hallucinations, heart block, convulsions. Effects may be exacerbated by associated hypokalaemia	Digoxin-specific antibody fragments e.g. Digiband 38 mg (British Medical Association & Royal Pharmaceutical Society of Great Britain 1999). Lignocaine is used to treat arrhythmias. Heart block may require pacing. Convulsions may be treated by use of phenytoin. Where hypokalaemia is present Magnesium IV 8 mmol (4 mL of 50%) may be repeated after 10–15 min (Resuscitation Council (UK) 1998)
Opioids	Narcotic analgesic	Varying degrees of coma, respiratory depression, pinpoint pupils	Naloxone 0.8 mg IV. Close monitoring and repeat doses of naloxone as it has a

Table 7.2 (*contd*)

Drug/Toxin	Action	Effects of overdose	Management
			shorter duration of action than many opioids (British Medical Association & Royal Pharmaceutical Society of Great Britain 1999)
Theophylline	Bronchodilation by relaxation of the smooth muscle of the bronchial tree Theophylline has a narrow therapeutic range which means that there is only a small difference between the therapeutic dose and toxic dose (Trounce 1994)	Vomiting, agitation, restlessness, dilated pupils, sinus tachycardia, hypoglycaemia, haematemesis, supraventricular tachycardia, ventricular tachycardia, profound hypokalaemia	Empty the stomach with activated charcoal if the OD has presented within 2 h Hypokalaemia – IV potassium chloride infusion and monitor ECG Agitation and convulsions are controlled by diazepam (emulsion preferred) Severe tachycardia, hypokalaemia and hyperglycaemia may be reversed by the administration of propranolol provided that the patient is not asthmatic

Bradycardia

As can be seen by the protocol shown in Figure 7.5, when presented with a patient who has a bradycardia, the practitioner must ask

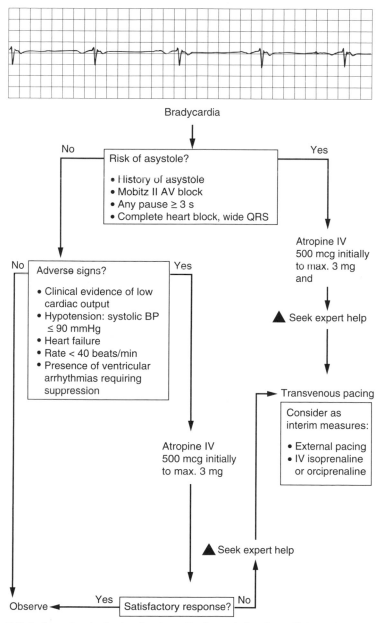

Fig. 7.5 Peri-arrest arrhythmias; bradycardia. Resusciation Council (UK) 1998, reproduced with permission.

1. Is there a risk of asystole? The nurse may be aware of the patient having a history of asystole either during this admission or prior admissions to hospital and this information needs to be conveyed to the medical team.

2. Are there any adverse signs? It is often the nursing staff who alert the medical staff to the change in the patient's status and in this would include any changes in blood pressure. The nurse should then make available the drugs that would be used in the protocol ready for when the physician arrives to see the patient.

Broad complex tachycardia

With this arrhythmia the practitioner is directed to ask the following questions:

1. Does the patient have a pulse? The most common cause of this type of arrhythmia is ventricular tachycardia. If the patient is pulseless then treat as for a VF/Pulseless VT arrest. If the patient has a pulse then the practitioner is directed to ask

2. Are there any adverse signs? As can be seen from the protocol, the interventions will depend on whether or not adverse signs are present (Fig. 7.6).

Narrow complex tachycardia

The commonest cause of this type of arrhythmia is supraventricular tachycardia. In the event of this arrhythmia occurring, the practitioner is directed towards trying vagal manoeuvres and/or intravenous adenosine (Resuscitation Council (UK) 1998).

Vagal manoeuvres are used to stimulate the vagus nerve in order to induce a reflex slowing of the heart. The most commonly used are carotid sinus massage or Valsalva manoeuvre.

Carotid sinus massage involves locating one of the carotid pulses and applying massage to that artery. This should not be used if the patient has been assessed as having a carotid bruit as it may result in rupture of a plaque that may embolize into the cerebral circulation and cause a cerebral vascular accident.

The Valsalva manoeuvre involves asking the patient to cough (forced expiration against a closed glottis) (Resuscitation Council (UK) 1998).

Adenosine is a component of the energy-rich compound adenosine triphosphate (ATP) and is given in an initial dose of 3 mg as a rapid bolus followed by a saline flush. If unsuccessful the dose can be repeated, doubling the dose each time up to 12 mg. Patients should be warned that they may experience transient unpleasant side-effects such as nausea, flushing and chest pain (British Medical Association & Royal Pharmaceutical Society of Great Britain 1999).

If these interventions are unsuccessful, then the next question asked is are there any adverse signs? The protocol then directs the physician as to what interventions may be used to correct the arrhythmia (Fig. 7.7).

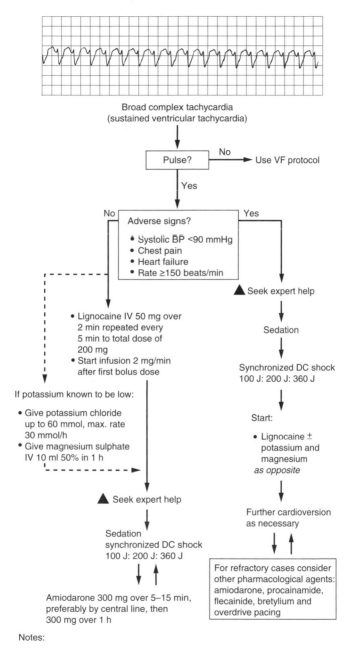

Fig. 7.6 Broad complex tachycardia. Resuscitation Council (UK) 1998, reproduced with permission.

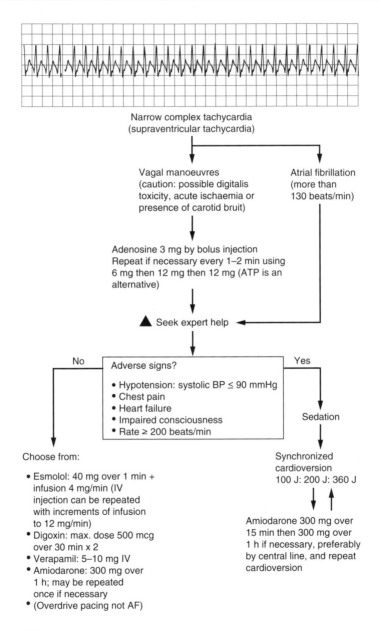

Narrow complex tachycardia
(supraventricular tachycardia)

Vagal manoeuvres
(caution: possible digitalis
toxicity, acute ischaemia or
presence of carotid bruit)

Atrial fibrillation
(more than
130 beats/min)

Adenosine 3 mg by bolus injection
Repeat if necessary every 1–2 min using
6 mg then 12 mg then 12 mg (ATP is an
alternative)

▲ Seek expert help ◄

No   Adverse signs?   Yes

• Hypotension: systolic BP ≤ 90 mmHg
• Chest pain
• Heart failure
• Impaired consciousness
• Rate ≥ 200 beats/min

Sedation

Choose from:

• Esmolol: 40 mg over 1 min +
  infusion 4 mg/min (IV
  injection can be repeated
  with increments of infusion
  to 12 mg/min)
• Digoxin: max. dose 500 mcg
  over 30 min x 2
• Verapamil: 5–10 mg IV
• Amiodarone: 300 mg over
  1 h; may be repeated
  once if necessary
• (Overdrive pacing not AF)

Synchronized
cardioversion
100 J: 200 J: 360 J

Amiodarone 300 mg over
15 min then 300 mg over
1 h if necessary, preferably
by central line, and repeat
cardioversion

Notes:

• Doses based on adult of average body weight
• In all cases give oxygen and establish IV access

Fig. 7.7 Narrow complex tachycardia. Resuscitation Council (UK) 1998, reproduced with permission.

CONCLUSION

Acknowledgement must be made that resuscitation attempts often occur in hospitals as an end-stage event when the patient has deteriorated to the point where resuscitation is required. In hospital, cardiopulmonary arrests are predictable events (Resuscitation Council (UK) 1998). Many patients who have reached this stage have poor organ reserve owing to either their pathologies or ageing processes. It is not surprising, therefore, that the current success rates for resuscitation attempts in hospital are poor (see chapter 8). It is vitally important therefore, that nurses develop their knowledge and skills in recognizing those patients whose pathologies may lead to cardiorespiratory arrest. On recognizing signs of deterioration in these patients, the nurse is responsible for alerting the medical team in order to ensure swift intervention to prevent cardiorespiratory arrest occurring.

In the event of the cardiac arrest, the nurse must know how to recognize and initiate both BLS and ALS protocols. At the beginning of the resuscitation event, the nurse may well take the role of team leader in the absence of a suitably trained physician and so it is important that nurses keep up to date with their skills and attend updates on resuscitation on at least a yearly basis. It is the role of the nurse to ensure that they maintain and improve professional knowledge and competence (UKCC 1992a).

Once the resuscitation team arrives, it is usual for the most senior attending physician to lead the resuscitation attempt, although it is not unknown for the resuscitation training officer or senior members of nursing staff to undertake this role (see chapter 4 for other aspects of the nurse's role).

The key to successful resuscitation is early identification (see chapter 6) and early intervention. The resuscitation team must work together to achieve a coordinated and efficient resuscitation attempt. It is to this end that the Resuscitation Council (UK) has created comprehensive training programmes aimed at any member of the health professions who might be involved in resuscitation attempts. It is recommended that nurses who are working in clinical areas caring for patients at high risk of cardiac arrest, should attend an ALS course and update those certificates on a 3–yearly basis.

Nurses are not just involved in the resuscitation attempt itself. The nurse in charge of the ward also has the responsibility of contacting and supporting relatives (see chapter 5). It must not be forgotten that there are other patients on the ward/unit who need continued observation and care (see chapter 4).

Once the resuscitation attempt has ended the nurse has the responsibility of attending to the patient and relatives (whether the attempt was successful or not; see chapter 5) and organizing the transfer of the patient (if appropriate). Documentation of the arrest is made in the case notes by the physician and in the nursing records by the nursing staff.

Collection of data to evaluate the resuscitation protocols has been recommended by the Resuscitation Council. The advisory statements made by the Resuscitation Council in 1997 recommended the collection of data in a systematic format using the Utstein template to ensure uniformity and comparability of data (see chapter 8). Ethical issues have limited the use of human subjects in research on resuscitation. Therefore, a systematic approach to the collection of data on resuscitation and its outcomes is the only way of developing a research base for future practice. Although some Trusts may have devised their own tools to audit resuscitation attempts, the Utstein template must be recommended in order to evaluate the effectiveness of the guidelines.

Advisory statements made by the Resuscitation Council in 1992 recommend the appointment of resuscitation training officers, often nurses, who have to complete courses for trainers, validated by the Resuscitation Council (UK) to carry out this important role in teaching a standardized and systematic approach to resuscitation.

REFERENCES

Abramson N S, Safar P, Sutton-Tyrrel K 1995 A randomised clinical trial of escalating doses of high dose epinephrine during cardiac resuscitation (abstract). Critical Care Medicine 23:A178

Adgey A A J, Devlin J E, Webb S W, Mulholland H 1982 Initiation of ventricular fibrillation outside hospital in patients with acute ischaemic heart disease. British Heart Journal 47:55–61

Advanced Life Support Group 1993 Advanced cardiac life support, the practical approach. Chapman & Hall, London

Alexander M F, Fawcett J N, Runciman P J (eds) 1994 Nursing practice in hospital and home: the adult. Churchill Livingstone, London

Bear P G, Myers J L 1994 Adult health nursing, 2nd edn. Mosby, London

Bossaert L (ed.) 1998 European Resuscitation Council guidelines for resuscitation. Elsevier Science, Amsterdam

Brimacombe J R, Berry A 1995 The incidence of aspiration associated with the laryngeal mask airway: a meta-analysis of published literature. Clinical Journal of Anaesthesia 7:297–305

British Medical Association and the Royal Pharmaceutical Society of Great Britain 1999 British national formulary. No 37. Bath Press, Avon

Bruce-Jones J 1997 The new guidelines. Nursing Standard 11(33):21–24

Caparelli E V, Chow M S S, Kluger J, Feildman A 1989 Difference in systematic and myocardial blood acid–base status during cardiopulmonary resuscitation. Critical Care Medicine 17:442–446

Cadwell G, Millar G, Quinn E, Vincent R, Chamberlain D A 1985 Simple mechanical methods for cardioversion: defence of precordial thump. British Medical Journal 291:627–630

Chamberlain D A, Cummins R O 1997 Advisory statements of the International Liaison Committee on Resuscitation (ILCOR). Resuscitation 34:99–100

Chamberlain D A, Bossaert L, Carli P, et al. 1992 A statement by the Advanced Life Support Working Party of the European Resuscitation Council. Resuscitation 24:111–121

Cobbe S M, Redmond M J, Watson J M, Hollingsworth J, Carrington D J 1991 'Heartstart Scotland' – initial experience of a national scheme for out of hospital defibrillation. British Medical Journal 302:1517–1520

Cummings R O, Chamberlain D A, Hazinski M F et al. 1997 Recommended guidelines for uniform reporting of data from in-hospital resuscitation. The in-hospital 'Utstein style'. Resuscitation 34:151–183

Deluna A B, Courrel P, Ledercq J F 1989 Ambulatory sudden cardiac death: mechanisms of production of fatal arrhythmia on the basis of data from 157 cases. American Heart Journal 117:151–159

Dorain P, Fain E S, Davey J M, Wrinkle R A 1986 Lidocaine causes a reversible, concentration-dependent increase in defibrillation energy requirements. Journal of the American College of Cardiology 8:327–332

Dowdle J R 1996 Ventricular standstill and cardiac percussion. Resuscitation 32:31–32

Ekstrom L, Herlitz J, Wennerblom B, Axelsson A, Bang A, Holmberg S 1994 Survival after cardiac arrest outside hospital over a 12 year period in Gothenburg. Resuscitation 27:181–188

European Resuscitation Council 1992 Guidelines for advanced life support. A statement by the Advanced Working Party of the European Resuscitation Council. Resuscitation 24:111–121

European Resuscitation Council Working Party 1993 Adult advanced life support: the European Resuscitation Council Guidelines1992, abridged. British Medical Journal 306(6892):1589–1592

Hapnes S A, Robertson C 1992 CPR – Drug delivery routes and systems: a Statement for the Advanced Life Support Working Party of the European Resuscitation Council. Resuscitation 24·137–142

Hardman J G (ed.) 1996 Goodman and Gilman's the pharmacological basis for therapentics, 9th edn. McGraw Hill, New York

Hargenten K M, Steuven H A, Waite E M et al. 1990 Per hospital experience with defibrillation of coarse ventricular fibrillation: a ten year review. Annals of Emergency Medicine 19:157–162

Herlitz J, Ekstrom L, Wennerblom B, Axelsson A, Bang A, Holmberg S 1995a Adrenaline in out of hospital ventricular fibrillation. Does it make any difference? Resuscitation 29:195–201

Herlitz J, Ekstrom L, Wennerblom B, Axelsson A, Bang A, Holmberg S 1995b Survival among patients with out of hospital cardiac arrest found in electromechanical dissociation. Resuscitation 29:97–106

ILCOR 1997 Special resuscitation situations; an advisory statement on conditions which may require modification in resuscitation procedures or techniques prepared by members of the International Liaison Committee on Resuscitation. Resuscitation 34:129–149

Kette F, Weil M H, Gazmuri R J, Bisera J, Rackow E C 1993 Intramyocardial hypercarbic acidosis during cardiac arrest and resuscitation. Critical Care Medicine 21:901–906

Kloeck W, Cummings R, Chamberlain D et al. 1997 The universal ALS algorithm: an advisory statement by the Advanced Life Support Working Group of the International Liaison Committee on Resuscitation. Resuscitation 34:109–111

Lake C L, Kron IL, Mentzer R M, Crampton R S 1986 Lidocaine enhances intraoperative ventricular defibrillation. Anesthesia and Analgesia 65:337–346

Larsen M P, Eisenberg M S, Cummins R O, Hallstrom A P 1993 Predicting survival from out-of-hospital cardiac arrest: a graphic model. Annals of Emergency Medicine 22:1652–1658

McCance K L, Huether S E 1994 Pathophysiology. The biological basis for disease in adults and children, 2nd edn. Mosby, London

Mapin DR, Brown CG, Dzuoncyk R 1991 Frequency analysis of the human and swine electrocardiogram during ventricular fibrillation. Resuscitation 22:85–91

Mattson-Porth C 1998 Pathophysiology – concepts of altered health states, 5th edn. Lippincott, Philadelphia

Natale A, Jones D L, Kim Y-H, Klein G J 1991 Effects of lidocaine on defibrillation threshold in the pig: evidence of anesthesia related increase. PACE 14: 1239–1244

Neumar R W, Brown C G, Robintaille P M, Altschuld R A 1990 Myocardial high energy phosphate metabolism during ventricular fibrillation with total circulatory arrest. Resuscitation 19(3):199–226

Nolan J, Smith G, Evans R, McCusker K, Lubas P, Parr M, Baskett P, members of the UK advisory ACD study group 1998 The United Kingdom pre hospital study of active compression–decompression resuscitation. Resuscitation 37:119–125

Owens T M, Robertson P, Twomey C, Doyle M, McDonald N, McShane A J 1995 The incidence of gastro-oesophageal reflux with the laryngeal mask. Anesthesia and Analgesia 80(5): 980–984, p. 88

Redding J S, Pearson J W 1963a Evaluation of drugs for cardiac resuscitation. Anaesthesiology 24:137–142

Redding J S, Pearson J W 1963b Adrenaline in cardiac resuscitation. American Heart Journal 66:210–214

Resuscitation Council (UK) 1998 Advanced life support course provider manual, 3rd edn. Resuscitation Council (UK), London

Reynolds E F 1993 Martindale. The extra pharmacopoeia. Pharmaceutical Press, London

Robertson C 1992 The precordial thump and cough techniques in advanced life support. Resuscitation 24:133–135

Robertson C, Steen P, Adgey J et al. 1998 The European Resuscitation Council guidelines for adult advanced life support. Resuscitation 37:81–90

Roth R, Stewart R D, Rogers K, Cannon G M 1984 Out of hospital cardiac arrest: factors associated with survival. Annals of Emergency Medicine 13:237–243

Rutter K M 1995 Tension pneumothorax: how to restore normal breathing. Nursing 25(4): 33

Sabin H I, Coghill S B, Khunti K, McNeill G O 1983 Accuracy of intracardiac injections determined by a post mortem study. Lancet 2(8358):1054–1055

Sedgewick M L, Dalziel K, Watson J, Carrington D J , Cobbe S M 1994 The causative rhythm in out of hospital cardiac arrests witnessed by the emergency medical services in the Heartstart Scotland project. Resuscitation 27: 55–59

Steedman D J, Robertson C E 1992 Acid base changes in arterial and central blood during cardiopulmonary resuscitation. Archives of Emergency Medicine 9: 169–176

Steill I G, Herbert P C, Weizman B W et al. 1992 High dose epinephrine in adult cardiac arrest. New England Journal of Medicine 327:1045–1050

Tang W, Weil M H, Gazmuri R J, Sun S, Duggal C, Bisera J 1991 Pulmonary ventilation/perfusion defects induced by epinephrine during cardiopulmonary resuscitation. Circulation 84(5):2101–2107

Tang W, Weil M H, Sun S, Marko N, Yang L, Gazmuri R J 1995 Epinephrine increases the severity of postresuscitation myocardial dysfunction. Circulation 92(10):3089–3093

Thelan L A, Davie J K, Urden L D, Lough M E 1994 Critical care nursing, diagnosis and management, 2nd edn. Mosby, London

Tortolani A J, Risucci D A, Rosati R J, Dixon R 1990 In hospital cardiopulmonary resuscitation; patient arrest and resuscitation factors associated with survival. Resuscitation 20:115–128

Trounce J 1994 Clinical pharmacology for n irses, 14th edn. Churchill Livingstone, Edinburgh, p. 83

Tunstall-Pedoe H, Bailey L, Chamberlain D, Marsden A, Ward M, Zideman D 1992 Survey of 3765 cardiopulmonary resuscitations in British hospitals (the BRESUS study). British Medical Journal 304:1347–1351

UKCC 1992a Code of Professional Conduct, 3rd edn. UKCC, London

UKCC 1992b Standards for the Administration of Medicines. UKCC, London

Weisfeldt M L, Kerber R E, McGoldrick R P et al. 1995 Public access defibrillation. A statement for healthcare professionals from the American Heart Association task force on automated enteral defibrillation. Circulation 92:2763

Woodhouse S P, Cox S, Boyd P, Case C, Weber M 1995 High-dose and standard dose adrenaline do not alter survival compared with placebo, in cardiac arrest. Resuscitation 30:243–249

Outcomes

Clive Weston

■ CONTENTS

INTRODUCTION

At first sight the outcome from an attempted resuscitation from cardiac arrest seems clear enough: the victim either lives or dies. It may appear entirely academic to develop an interest in outcomes, rather than in the management of an individual patient. However, the end of the 1990s is a time that sees increased emphasis on outcomes. The measurement and publication of the effects of medical interventions is becoming ubiquitous in the provision of health care.

WHY STUDY OUTCOMES?

Part of this move towards 'Outcomes Research' stems from a desire to increase accountability of, and therefore control over, health professionals and to compare different clinical interventions with respect to cost and effect. There are a number of other relevant issues (see Box 8.1). Not only is

---

Box 8.1 Usefulness of outcome measurement

- Comparison between centres
- Comparison of resuscitation techniques
- Audit standards
- Informing 'Do Not Resuscitate' order
- Predicting survival
- Increased accountability
- Confirming the efficacy of surrogate outcome measures.

a measurement of outcome a necessary component of research, it allows a comparison to be made between centres that use similar, or different, resuscitation techniques, between different systems and between different times. A caveat is that like is compared with like, or at least that allowances are made for case-mix. When a significant variation in outcomes is encountered that cannot be explained by differences in case-mix, an analysis of the process of resuscitation may provide an indicator to the cause of the variation. Outcome measures may also provide the standards against which performance can be measured during audit.

Measuring outcome is also important in recognizing the limitation of resuscitation. Successful resuscitation is still the exception, yet it is falsely represented in the media, where the majority of actors survive episodes of 'cardiac arrest' (Diem *et al.* 1996). Realistic expectations are important for rescuers and the relatives of victims. False expectations lead to despondency, disappointment, guilt and blame. By measuring outcomes, factors associated with good or bad results can be identified. This leads to an ability to predict recovery following cardiac arrest and the ability to determine where attempts to resuscitate would be futile. This is important both in the development of 'do not resuscitate' orders and in the management of cardiac arrests outside hospital (Marsden *et al.* 1995).

WHICH OUTCOMES SHOULD BE MEASURED?

The goal of resuscitation is to return the patient to their pre-arrest state both physically and neurologically. This recovery should be maintained in the long term. Thus, outcome can be expressed in terms of survival (alive or dead?), longevity (alive for how long?) and quality (how well did the patient live?).

The literature on resuscitation has been characterized by wide variations in nomenclature that have made interpretation and comparison very difficult. This has been likened to a 'tower of Babel' of articles (Eisenberg *et al.* 1990). There has even been lack of agreement on what constitutes the outcome. In some studies, a 'save' or 'successful resuscitation' has been defined as a return of spontaneous circulation (for as little as 20 min), in others as admission to a hospital ward (following pre-hospital arrest) and in others as discharge from hospital. Relatively few reports have included information on the cerebral status of survivors or on long-term survival. There may be arguments in favour of using any number of these outcomes. For example, an ambulance service may feel that its responsibility stops once a patient arrives at a hospital and that the most important outcome is the viability of the patient at this time. Subsequent management within the hospital may have effects on the later outcome and is beyond the control of the emergency services. In the same way, members of a hospital cardiac arrest team may believe that an assessment of their performance should be based on the survival of the patient at the end of the initial resuscitation attempt rather than the status of the patient 1 week, 1 month or 1 year later.

A hospital manager may look on successful discharge from hospital following a cardiac arrest as the most important outcome, particularly when this is linked with length of stay and intensive care bed-usage. It could be argued that only the victim and their relatives would be interested in the outcome of long-term good quality survival.

Weston *et al.* (1997a) collected data from 954 attempted resuscitations from pre-hospital cardiorespiratory arrest and reported outcomes of 14.3% for admission to hospital, and 7.1% for discharge home. A smaller study of in-hospital resuscitation in an American cancer centre reported a rate of return of spontaneous circulation of 66.3%, with only 9.6% patients surviving to hospital discharge and 3.6% surviving to 1 year (Varon *et al.* 1998). The total in-hospital charges for those 52 patients who had return of spontaneous circulation was about 2.9 million US dollars.

In the same way that there are numerous definitions of a successful outcome, there are also many possible ways of defining a case of cardiac arrest. Variations in the definition of a case lead to differences in the denominator when calculating survival rates. For example, Eisenberg *et al.* (1993), using the same data set of out-of-hospital cardiac arrest victims, reported survival rates of 18% when the denominator included the whole data set and up to 49% where the denominator was restricted to patients whose arrests were witnessed, where the initial rhythm on arrival of the ambulance service was ventricular fibrillation (VF), where bystanders initiated cardiopulmonary resuscitation (CPR) within 4 min and where definitive advanced life support (ALS) was available within 8 min.

One final difficulty in comparing outcomes relates to differences in the methodology of data collection. Within hospital practice there is perhaps a little more uniformity, but even here there are likely to be significant differences in recorded details – for example, where data collection depends on retrospective completion of cardiac arrest forms compared with an interview of the arrest team by a researcher or even video tape recordings of the actual arrest. Outside hospital, direct contact with the ambulance crew significantly increases the proportion of arrests that are designated as witnessed VF (i.e. when the arrest develops in the presence of the ambulance crew) when compared with retrospective analysis of completed despatch forms (Gallagher *et al.* 1994). Perhaps the most accurate data collection system would involve investigators observing directly the resuscitation. While some resuscitation-training officers attempt to do this within hospital, very few pre-hospital services have used this method (Waalewijn *et al.* 1998).

SURROGATE MARKERS OF OUTCOME

When aspects of training or provision of resuscitation services can be shown to predict improved survival they can be used as proxy or surrogate markers of outcome. This is a useful concept. Such factors could include the response time of a cardiac arrest team or emergency medical service, the interval from collapse to the first defibrillation or (perhaps) the presence of a paramedic at the scene of an out-of-hospital arrest (see below). Since the quality of basic life support (BLS) influences survival (Wik *et al.* 1994), a variety of methods for assessing the acquisition and retention of resuscitation skills have been developed and may serve as surrogate markers of outcome (Berden *et al.* 1992, Lester *et al.* 1997). Assessments of advanced cardiac life support (ACLS) skills may also be used (Kaye *et al.* 1990).

The weakness of all these measures is that they address only one component, or a limited number of components that combine to affect outcome and, in certain circumstances, may have less influence than expected. For example, the demonstration that ALS skills are optimum may be of little value if response times are prolonged. Moreover, merely providing ACLS training and using the number of doctors trained to this level has not been shown to improve overall outcome (Kaye 1995). Wherever possible, measures of true outcome (however defined) should be the goal.

UNIFORM REPORTING OF DATA – THE UTSTEIN STYLE

There is still no 'gold standard' methodology for investigating the incidence management and outcome of cardiorespiratory arrest. However, difficulties in the reporting of data (numerators and denominators) have been addressed. Members of a variety of organizations interested in resuscitation attended a meeting at Utstein Abbey near Stavanger, Norway, in 1990 to discuss such problems. At a second meeting, a report was drafted that focused on out-of-hospital cardiac arrest and included a glossary of terms, a template for reporting data, a recommendation for the description of emergency medical systems and a variety of definitions of time intervals, clinical items and outcomes. This system of reporting data was labelled 'the Utstein style' (Chamberlain *et al.* 1991). More recently, a similar set of guidelines designed for in-hospital resuscitation has been published, and with it a standard report form for data collection (Cummins *et al.* 1997). Other guidelines exist for reporting outcomes of paediatric resuscitation (Zaritsky *et al.* 1995) and experimental (laboratory-based) resuscitation (Idris *et al.* 1996). Although revision of the original Utstein definitions is bound to occur, the concept of displaying results in template format will undoubtedly persist. For out-of-hospital resuscitation, this type of display has been used in reports from a variety of centres (Kuisma & Maatta 1996, Weston *et al.* 1997b, Kette *et al.* 1998). The template consists of a number of boxes arranged rather like a family tree. The first box defines the population, for example the total number of hospital inpatients over a given time or the population served by an emergency ambulance service. Later boxes contain various pre-specified subsets of patients. The number at each level serves as the numerator for the box above and the denominator for the box below. In this way, multiple outcomes, expressed as rates, can be calculated. A gold standard outcome has been defined for out-of-hospital cardiac arrest: this is the number of individuals discharged alive from hospital, divided by the number of those whose pre-hospital cardiac arrest was witnessed, was of cardiac aetiology and who were in ventricular fibrillation when cardiac rhythm was first assessed. No gold standard outcome has yet been agreed for in-hospital resuscitation, although the percentage of those surviving until hospital discharge and of those alive at 1 year would seem important rates to report.

The Utstein task force also suggested that results could be expressed in terms of the number of attempted resuscitations, the number of initial survivors, the number surviving 24 h, or the number leaving hospital alive, for each survivor alive at 1 year.

The same group also emphasized the importance of assessment of quality of life in reporting outcome but were unable to define a standard instrument for its measurement. As a minimum, they recommended recording the time to awakening (Longstreth *et al.* 1983), the immediate Glasgow Coma Scale and subsequent cerebral performance category (CPC) at discharge and at later review.

PREDICTION OF OUTCOME

As mentioned above, one reason to measure outcome is to describe factors associated either with a good or bad outcome and to develop the ability to predict the likelihood that an individual can survive an episode of cardiac arrest. Such factors include characteristics of the patient (age, gender, social class, racial group and previous medical history), details of the arrest (place of collapse, presence of a witness, aetiology and initial rhythm) and characteristics of the resuscitation attempt (the initiator of BLS, delays to treatment and the availability of ALS skills). Many series in the literature have analysed these variables and reported their association with a successful outcome. The simplest way of presenting this association has been to use univariate analysis. Here the frequency of one particular variable is compared between those with a good outcome and those with a bad outcome. This comparison is made in isolation and does not take into account any other variable. However, the variables themselves are associated and there may be many interactions between variables. Multivariate analysis seeks to adjust for these interactions and uses statistical methods to define the relative importance of numerous variables and to identify those variables that are independently predictive of survival. For example, using univariate analysis to describe a data set of victims of pre-hospital cardiac arrest, discharge from hospital was more likely if the collapse was witnessed, if bystanders initiated CPR, if the patient was in ventricular fibrillation and when CPR and ACLS were provided promptly (Weston *et al.* 1997b). Analysing the same data set using multivariate analysis confirmed the importance of any delay from collapse to the initiation of CPR and to the provision of ACLS, but suggested that the provision of bystander-initiated CPR was a marker for early CPR (Weston *et al.* 1997a). The fact that CPR was started early was more relevant than who was responsible for providing it. Again, univariate analysis has shown poorer survival rates in older patients, yet they are more likely to have unwitnessed arrests and are more likely to be found in asystole. These last two factors are themselves associated with a poorer outcome (Bonnin *et al.* 1993).

The same is true within hospital. Using a data set of approximately 800 in-hospital cardiac arrests, Cooper & Cade (1997) used univariate analysis to show a significant survival benefit for those patients arresting within the coronary care unit (CCU) compared with those arresting in other areas. A survival benefit was also shown in those who had been admitted to hospital because of cardiac disease rather than any other cause. Clearly, these two factors interact: patients admitted with cardiac disease are more likely to be placed in a CCU than other patients. Moreover, when logistic regression (multivariate) analysis was performed these two factors (arrests in CCU, admission with cardiac disease) were no longer significantly associated with outcome and had been subsumed by more predictive factors, such as the rhythm of the arrest and the speed with which resuscitation was performed.

For both in-hospital and out-of-hospital cardiac arrest, a number of predictive models have been devised to describe the likelihood of survival. A model based on the Seattle database of out-of-hospital cardiac arrest suggested a 67% survival rate if CPR, defibrillation and ALS could be delivered at the time of collapse. There is an absolute reduction in survival of 2.3%/min delay before CPR (with additional/concurrent reductions of 1.1%/min delay before defibrillation and 2.1%/min delay before ACLS) (Larsen *et al.* 1993). Others have developed a 'survival index' based on a mathematical equation that combines the amplitude of ventricular fibrillation and the number of base-line crossings of VF per second, together with the age of the patient (Monsieurs *et al.* 1998).

Similar predictive tools have been developed for in-hospital cardiac arrest. For example, a prognostic index was developed combining the rhythm of the arrest, performance of intubation or defibrillation, the delay to defibrillation and the age of the patient (Marwick *et al.* 1991). However, even sophisticated models fail to be totally accurate in predicting outcome and they are certainly not sophisticated enough to do anything other than form the basis for discussions on resuscitation status (Ebell *et al.* 1997).

FACTORS ASSOCIATED WITH SURVIVAL

Notwithstanding the problems discussed above relating to the definition of 'a case' and 'successful resuscitation' and bearing in mind the importance of multivariate analysis, numerous factors are described in the literature to be associated with survival. These are listed for both out-of-hospital and in-hospital resuscitation in Boxes 8.2 and 8.3, respectively. The significance of these factors varies from one report to another, although the common

Box 8.2 Factors associated with outcome of out-of-hospital arrests

	Good outcome	Poor outcome
Patient factors	Higher social class Absence of co-morbidity	Very elderly or infants Lower social classes Significant co-morbidity
Arrest variables	Witnessed arrest Arrest witnessed by ambulance personnel Initial rhythm VF Primary respiratory arrest Arrest in street	Unwitnessed arrest Arrest at home Initial rhythm asystole or EMD
Resuscitation variables	Bystander CPR Good quality CPR Early CPR (<1 min) Early defibrillation Return of circulation at scene	Delayed CPR (4 min+) Poor-quality CPR Delayed defibrillation No return of circulation on arrival at hospital

Box 8.3 Factors associated with outcome of in-hospital arrests

	Good outcome	Poor outcome
Patient factors	Absence of severe co-morbidity Acute coronary syndromes	Presence of malignancy, end-stage organ failure The very elderly
Arrest variables	Initial rhythm VF/VT Primary respiratory arrest Witnessed arrest Arrest in CCU	Initial rhythm asystole or EMD Unwitnessed arrest Arrest in general ward
Resuscitation variables	Short duration CPR Immediate CPR Early defibrillation	Prolonged CPR Delayed CPR Delayed defibrillation or defibrillation inappropriate

thread running through virtually all reports is the importance of the primary arrhythmia when the arrest begins, the rhythm present when resuscitation starts, the provision of prompt BLS and early defibrillation (when this is appropriate). For in-hospital arrest, pre-existing patient factors are particularly important. With respect to survival to discharge following in-hospital cardiac arrest, most of the variation between studies is explained in terms of the specific patient populations involved (Ballew & Philbrick 1995). Therefore, survival is better when cardiac arrest complicates acute myocardial infarction occurring in otherwise healthy individuals, compared with arrests occurring in those with multisystem failure.

While there are still plenty of new avenues for research, it is important to remember that two specific interventions that could intuitively be assumed to lead to a better outcome have, to date, failed to be linked conclusively to survival. For in-hospital resuscitation, much effort is being put into the systematic training of medical and nursing staff in ACLS skills. Few studies have been able to demonstrate an association between such training and improvements in survival (Cooper & Cade 1997). Even these studies have not been able to differentiate between defibrillator skills and other ALS skills. In out-of-hospital cardiac arrest, paramedic skills (other than defibrillation) have anecdotally been reported as essential for successful outcome (Weston & Stephens 1992). However, larger British studies disagree about the added benefit of paramedics. Mitchell *et al.* (1997) showed no added benefit, whereas a review of 1547 pre-hospital cardiac arrests in Nottinghamshire suggested that the presence of a paramedic did lead to significant improvement in outcome (Soo *et al.* 1999).

BRITISH RESULTS

For out-of-hospital cardiac arrest, the best reported survival rate (to discharge from hospital) from any large series is 49%. This was achieved by American paramedics in a select group of patients whose arrests were witnessed, where the initial rhythm on arrival of the ambulance service was ventricular fibrillation, where bystanders initiated CPR within 4 min and where definitive ALS was available within 8 min (Eisenberg *et al.* 1993). British centres have reported far lower survival rates. In the largest Welsh series, an ambulance service with both paramedic and non-paramedic vehicles reported an overall survival rate of 6.8%. In the subset of patients whose arrests were of cardiac aetiology, witnessed by a bystander and who were in ventricular fibrillation, 21% were admitted to hospital and 13% were discharged (Weston *et al.* 1997b). Similarly, in a study of the Scottish ambulance service, providing emergency care with non-paramedic vehicles equipped with a defibrillator, the same subset had an 11% discharge rate (Sedgwick *et al.* 1993). When ambulance personnel were present at the time of arrest the discharge rate was 33% in Wales and 38% in Scotland. In the largest English series, 14.3% of patients were admitted to hospital and 6.1% were discharged. However, in the subset that was in ventricular fibrillation, 11.7% left hospital alive (Soo *et al.* 1999).

Results for in-hospital resuscitation are even more variable and, as mentioned above, much of this variation can be related to differences in the patient population studied, as well as to the usual problems with case definitions. In a review of 68 studies, Ballew & Philbrick (1995) found survival to discharge from hospital ranging from 0 to 28.9%. The British studies included in their review had results ranging from 8.7 to 21.9%. An earlier review of 42 papers and almost 13 000 cases showed an average 24-h survival rate of 39% and a discharge rate of 15% (McGrath 1987). The largest British multicentred study, including results from over 3500 cardiac arrests predominantly beginning within hospital, reported an immediate survival rate of 45%, a 24-h survival of 32% and a discharge survival of 21% (Tunstall-Pedoe et al. 1992). These results were very similar to the largest single-centred British series of 808 arrests, which reported immediate survival of 43%, a 24-h survival of 30% and a discharge survival of 22% (Cooper & Cade 1997).

COST OF SUCCESSFUL RESUSCITATION

Mention has already been made above of the high cost (US$2.9 million) incurred by 52 patients with cancer who had been successfully resuscitated following in-hospital cardiac arrest (Varon et al. 1998). Surprisingly few centres have reported any data regarding the cost of any aspect of resuscitation, such as training, equipment, delivery of care and post-resuscitation care. An early report from Sweden, using prices in 1982, sought to estimate the total cost in providing care for 277 out-of-hospital arrest victims, of which 28 were admitted to the hospital wards and nine were discharged. Of the total costs, 12% were attributable to training and equipping the emergency medical service and the remaining 88% related to hospital costs. At 1982 prices, the total cost per life saved was approximately US$14 700 (Jakobsson et al. 1987). Ebell & Kruse (1994) devised a model for costing cardio-pulmonary resuscitation. Using an average survival rate of 12.8%, they estimated a cost of US$110 270/survivor of in-hospital cardiac arrest and a cost of US$61 000/quality-adjusted life year. This compared well with US$64 000/quality-adjusted life year in the management of symptomatic single-vessel coronary disease in patients with angina. Finally, Lee et al. (1996) performed a MEDLINE search using the categories 'cardio-pulmonary resuscitation' and 'cost'. Basing their assessment on previous data discovered in this way, they estimated the cost per 6-month survivor to range from US$344 314 to US$966 759 in 1995 and the cost per quality-adjusted life year to range from US$191 286 to US$537 088. This was based on a projection of approximately 20% survival to hospital admission following out-of-hospital cardiac arrest and approximately 5% survival to 6 months.

CONCLUSION

In summary, the study of outcomes following cardiac arrest is most important. Resuscitation practice should be firmly based on evidence of the best possible outcome obtained from methodically sound research. Even where research is not the primary aim, accurate data collection of cardiac arrest and outcome is mandatory.

Comparisons between units will best be achieved using a uniform system of data collection, utilizing agreed definitions of numerators and denominators, namely the Utstein style of reporting. Nurses are involved in all stages of resuscitation within hospital, from advising on 'do not resuscitate' notices, calling the arrest team, initiating BLS, performing defibrillation, to post-arrest management of relatives and patients. The final recording of reliable data relating to process and outcome is an equally important, although less glamorous aspect of the role of all those involved in cardiac arrest management.

REFERENCES

Ballew K A, Philbrick J T 1995 Causes of variation in reported in-hospital CPR survival: a critical review. Resuscitation 30:203–215

Berden H J J M, Pijls N H J, Willems F F, Hendrick J M A, Crul J F 1992 A scoring system for basic cardiac life support skills in training situations. Resuscitation 23:21–23

Bonnin M J, Pepe P E, Clark P S 1993 Survival in the elderly after out-of-hospital cardiac arrest. Critical Care Medicine 21:1645–1651

Chamberlain D A, Cummings R O, Abramson N et al. 1991 Recommended guidelines for uniform reporting of data from out-of-hospital cardiac arrest: the 'Utstein style'. Resuscitation 22:1–26

Cooper S, Cade J 1997 Predicting survival, in-hospital cardiac arrests: resuscitation survival variables and training effectiveness. Resuscitation 35:17–22

Cummins R O, Chamberlain D A, Hazinski M F et al. 1997 Recommended guidelines for reviewing, reporting, and conducting research on in-hospital resuscitation: the in-hospital 'Utstein style'. Resuscitation 34:151–183

Diem S J, Lantos J D, Tulsky J A 1996 Cardiopulmonary resuscitation on television. Miracles and misinformation. New England Journal of Medicine 334:1578–1582

Ebell M H, Kruse J A 1994 A proposed model for the cost of cardiopulmonary resuscitation. Medical Care 32:640–649

Ebell M H, Kruse J A, Smith M, Novak J, Draderwilcox J 1997 Failure of three decision rules to predict the outcome of in-hospital cardiopulmonary resuscitation. Medical Decision Making 17:171–177

Eisenberg M S, Cummings R O, Damon S, Larsen M P, Hearne T R 1990 Survival rates from out-of-hospital cardiac arrest: recommendations for uniform definitions and data to report. Annals of Emergency Medicine 19: 1249–1259

Eisenberg M S, Cummins R O, Larsen M P 1993 Numerators, denominators, and survival rates: reporting survival from out-of-hospital cardiac arrest. American Journal of Emergency Medicine 9(6):544–546

Gallagher E J, Lombardi G, Gennis P, Treiber M 1994 Methodology-dependent variation in documentation of outcome predictors in out-of-hospital cardiac arrest. Academic Emergency Medicine 1:423–429

Idris A H, Becker L B, Ornato J P et al. 1996 Utstein-style guidelines for uniform reporting of laboratory CPR. Circulation 94:2324–2336

Jakobsson J, Nyquist O, Rehnquist N, Norberg K A 1987 Cost of a saved life following out-of-hospital cardiac arrest resuscitated by specially trained ambulance personnel. Acta Anaesthesiology Scandinavia 31:426–429

Kaye W 1995 Research in ACLS training – which methods improve skill and knowledge retention? Respiratory Care 40: 538–549

Kaye W, Wynne G, Marteau T, Dubin H G, Rallis S F, Simons R S, Evans T R 1990 An advanced resuscitation training course for pre-registration house officers. Journal of the Royal College of Physicians of London 24:51–54

Kette F, Sbrojavacca R, Rellini G et al. 1998 Epidemiology and survival rate of out-of-hospital cardiac arrest in north-east Italy: The FACS study. Resuscitation 36:1953–1959

Kuisma M, Maatta T 1996 Out-of-hospital cardiac arrests in Helsinki – Utstein style reporting. Heart 76:18-23

Larsen M P, Eisenberg M S, Cummins R O, Hallstrom A P 1993 Predicting survival from out-of-hospital cardiac arrest: a graphic model. Annals of Emergency Medicine 22:1652–1658

Lee K H, Angus D C, Abramson N S 1996 Cardiopulmonary resuscitation: what cost to cheat death? Critical Care Medicine 24:2046–2052

Lester C A, Morgan C L, Donnelly P D, Assar D 1997 Assessing with CARE: an innovative method of testing the approach and casualty assessment components of basic life support, using video recording. Resuscitation 34:43–49

Longstreth W T Jr, Diehr P, Inui T S 1983 Predication of awakening after out-of-hospital cardiac arrest. New England Journal of Medicine 308:1378–1382

Marsden A K, Ng G A, Dalziel K, Cobbe S M 1995 When is it futile for ambulance personnel to initiate cardiopulmonary resuscitation? British Medical Journal 311:49–51

Marwick T H, Case C C, Siskind V, Woodhouse S P 1991 Prediction of survival from resuscitation: a prognostic index derived from multivariate logistic model analysis. Resuscitation 22:129–137

McGrath R B 1987 In-house cardiopulmonary resuscitation after a quarter of a century. Annals of Emergency Medicine 16:1365–1368

Mitchell R G, Guly U M, Rainer T H, Robertson C E 1997 Can the full range of paramedic skills improve survival from out-of-hospital cardiac arrests? Journal of Accident and Emergency Medicine 14:274–277

Monsieurs K G, De Cauwer H, Wuyts F L, Bossaert L L 1998 A rule for early outcome classification of out-of-hospital cardiac arrest patients presenting with ventricular fibrillation. Resuscitation 36:37–44

Sedgwick M L, Dalziel K, Watson J, Carrington D J, Cobbe S M 1993 Performance of an established system of first-responder out-of-hospital defibrillation. The second year of the Heartstart Scotland Project in the 'Utstein Style'. Resuscitation 26:75–88

Soo L H, Gray D, Young T, Huff N, Skene A, Hampton J R 1999 Resuscitation from out-of-hospital cardiac arrest: is survival dependent on who is available at the scene? Heart 81:47–52

Tunstall-Pedoe H, Bailey L, Chamberlain D A, Marsden A K, Ward M E, Zideman D A 1992 Survey of 3765 cardiopulmonary resuscitations in British hospitals (the BRESUS Study): methods and overall results. British Medical Journal 304:1347–1351

Varon J, Walsh G L, Marik P E, Fromm R E 1998 Should a cancer patient be resuscitated following an in-hospital cardiac arrest? Resuscitation 36: 165–168

Waalewijn R A, de Vos R, Koster R W 1998 Out-of-hospital cardiac arrests in Amsterdam and its surrounding areas: results from the Amsterdam resuscitation study (ARREST) in Utstein style. Resuscitation 38:157–167

Weston C F M, Stephens M R 1992 An audit of cardiac arrest management by extended trained ambulance crew. Resuscitation 23:207–216

Weston C F M, Wilson R J, Jones S D 1997a Predicting survival from out-of-hospital cardiac arrest: a multivariate analysis. Resuscitation 34:27–34

Weston C F M, Jones S D, Wilson R J 1997b Outcome of out-of-hospital cardiorespiratory arrest in South Glamorgan. Resuscitation 34:227–233

Wik L, Steen P A, Bircher N G 1994 Quality of bystander cardiopulmonary
resuscitation influences outcome after pre-hospital cardiac arrest. Resuscitation
28:195–203

Zaritsky A, Nadkarni V, Hazinski M F *et al.* 1995 Recommended guidelines for
uniform reporting of paediatric advanced life support: the Paediatric Utstein Style.
Resuscitation 30:95–115

Airway management

Brian Stone

■ CONTENTS

Introduction
Anatomical principles
Airway management

Decompression of a tension
pneumothorax
Conclusion

INTRODUCTION

A number of advances have been made in the field of cardiopulmonary resuscitation (CPR) over the past decade, which have served to improve patient survival in both hospital and pre-hospital arrests. One of these, automated defibrillation, is recognized as a major step forward, enabling this treatment to be provided by a wider range of personnel in a variety of situations. On the administration side, the adoption of guidelines by the UK and European Resuscitation Councils has been a great advance in standardizing training and clinical application. This has resulted in cardiac arrest being more easily understood and better managed by health care professionals. One area of cardiopulmonary resuscitation that has not advanced appreciably since the introduction of the self-inflating bag in the mid 1960s and the pocket mask in the 1970s has been airway management.

All other skills in cardiopulmonary resuscitation are without purpose if we fail to manage the airway of patients effectively. Without a patent airway, there can be no breathing and hypoxic damage to the brain will ensue in spite of other measures. The assessment of the airway and its patency is therefore the priority in any circumstance. Patency of the airway and adequacy of ventilation is dependent on the equipment used and the level of training and retention of these skills of the first responder. Effective airway management is essentially a repertoire of practical skills, and these must be learned and practised, initially on manikins and subsequently on consented anaesthetized patients under skilled supervision. It might be said that there are problems in teaching effective airway bag/valve/mask ventilation skills (Stone *et al.* 1998) and considerable naivety in expecting health-care professionals to provide mouth-to-mouth ventilation in hospital (Stone *et al.* 1994). Although airway management is not the sole factor determining patient survival, incorrectly managed or wrongly applied, it can have needlessly disastrous consequences. A sound theoretical grasp of the techniques is important before practical training commences and it is the aim of this chapter to provide this knowledge; however, it is no substitute for practical training. It is therefore recommended that after reading this chapter, you should contact your local resuscitation training officer for practical training.

At the top end of the spectrum in airway management is the endotracheal tube, the undisputed 'gold standard'. However, correct insertion is a skill which can be difficult to acquire and even more difficult to maintain. Use of the endotracheal tube is usually limited to a small number of trained personnel who carry out the procedure frequently, such as anaesthetists in hospitals and paramedics in the community. Considerable delay can occur in obtaining a skilled intubator during in-hospital arrests, which occur at night.

It would appear that there is a gap between skilled intubation, which provides a patent airway and delivers oxygen solely to the lungs, and simpler methods of airway management, in which technique can be poor and oxygen or expired air can be directed both into the lungs and into the stomach. The laryngeal mask airway (LMA) fills the gap between the endotracheal tube and the facemask in anaesthesia. Its unique positioning over the laryngeal inlet offers a potential to fill the same gap in cardiopulmonary resuscitation. The LMA was first described by its inventor, Dr Archie Brain, in 1983 and was subsequently made available for general use in anaesthesia in 1985. Acceptance in this field has been rapid and more than 1000 papers and letters have been published world-wide, a number of which have proposed and reported its use in cardiopulmonary resuscitation (Davies et al. 1990, Stone et al. 1993)

ANATOMICAL PRINCIPLES

The airway is divided into two parts, the upper and lower airway. The upper airway extends from the mouth and nostrils, via the oral and nasal cavities over the back of the tongue to the pharynx, and from there to the larynx and vocal cords (Fig. 9.1). The lower airway is from the larynx to the alveoli via the bronchial tree.

Upper airway

The patency of the upper airway depends on two key factors:

- No physical obstruction or foreign body present
- No loss of neuromuscular control of the tongue.

Physical obstruction can be by anything from broken teeth, blood, vomit and thick sputum. While conscious or in normal sleep, the brain maintains the tone of the glossopharyngeal muscles which support the tongue and prevent it falling back to obstruct the airway. An unconscious patient will lose this control and pharyngeal blockage by the tongue results.

Lower airway

While small foreign bodies may pass into the larynx and obstruct a bronchus, they are less likely to be as immediately life-threatening as an

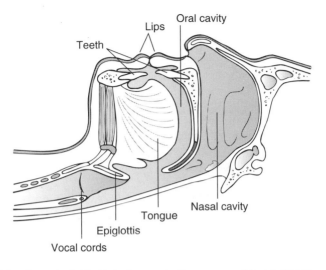

Teeth

Lips

Oral cavity

Vocal cords

Epiglottis

Tongue

Nasal cavity

Fig. 9.1 The airway is divided into two parts, the upper and lower airway.

upper airway obstruction. Lower airway obstruction can result from illness such as asthma, in which inflammatory exudate pours into the bronchi and the interstitial space causing oedema of the bronchial wall and worsening bronchospasm. Blood and vomit can obstruct the bronchial tree or it can be kinked by a tension pneumothorax, or compressed by mediastinal injury and swelling.

AIRWAY MANAGEMENT

Simple manoeuvres

Having ensured that the victim is safe to approach, the rescuer should 'shake and shout' to assess responsiveness. If the patient is unconscious, the rescuer shouts for help and then visually inspects for any obvious foreign body or vomit in the victim's mouth.

The head tilt–chin lift manoeuvre

The head tilt–chin lift manoeuvre is used (see also chapter 6) to open the patient's airway. This does not involve extending the cervical spine: the skull is tilted at the atlanto-occipital joint then the chin is lifted by grasping the victim's mandible. The effect of this technique is to lift the tongue, which is attached to the mandible, from the back of the pharynx (Fig. 9.2).

The jaw thrust

The jaw thrust is used in a patient who is of large build and thick set, or in whom you suspect a cervical spine injury. The head is stabilized with the balls of the rescuer's thumbs on the victim's maxillae, the middle fingers

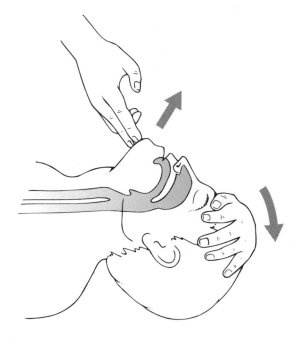

Fig. 9.2 The head tilt–chin lift manoeuvre.

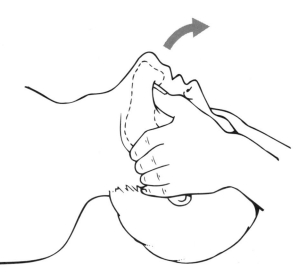

Fig. 9.3 The jaw thrust.

lift behind the angle of the mandible and the thumbs hold the patient's mouth open (Fig. 9.3). This can sometimes require considerable effort.

If unsuccessful, these manoeuvres must be attempted again, with more vigilance and effort. If a patent airway has still not been obtained, either there is a foreign body present or the rescuer's skills are inadequate, or perhaps there may be some physical anomaly in the patient's anatomy. In a victim of trauma, the control of the cervical spine is simultaneous with opening the airway, and only the jaw thrust should be used.

The Heimlich manoeuvre and abdominal thrusts

A patient who is choking will hold their throat and indicate that they are in distress. They will respond when asked if they are choking. They should be asked to cough and slaps to the back, between the shoulders, are applied with each cough. If the patient cannot cough, the rescuer stands behind them and places the clenched fist of one hand midway between the xiphisternum and the umbilicus. The other hand grips the fist and sharp inward and upward jerks are applied to the patient's abdomen. The idea is suddenly to push the diaphragm up into the chest, reducing intrathoracic volume, in effect producing an artificial cough to expel the obstruction. As the patient loses consciousness, they are allowed to sink to the floor and alternating chest compressions (as used in CPR) and abdominal thrusts are applied. The airway is continually inspected to check whether the obstruction has appeared to a point from which it can be retrieved. In infants, abdominal thrusts are not used because the relatively prominent liver, lying under the right costal margin, can be seriously damaged. These manoeuvres are continued in cycles until ventilation becomes possible.

Attempts may be made to ventilate the patient, once a patent airway has been secured. Although these manoeuvres are called simple, they are fundamental to airway management and are used in conjunction with the more advanced techniques that follow. Remember, death is final and we cannot go back and try again: the victim must have a patent airway to survive.

Advanced methods

The head tilt–chin lift and jaw thrust are the basic manoeuvres and they form part of the more advanced methods of airway management and ventilation of the apnoeic patient. It should be remembered that the availability of effective high-flow suction is a universal requirement of airway management and must always be available. Oxygen should also be used as soon as possible at high flow rates to achieve high inspired oxygen percentages in order to reduce the risk of cerebral hypoxia.

Airway adjuncts

The oropharyngeal airway (Guedel)

This is used in unconscious patients as an adjunct to the basic airway manoeuvres. It is inserted upside down, well-lubricated and rotated as it is passed over the tongue so that the tip lies in the oropharynx (Fig. 9.4). Its

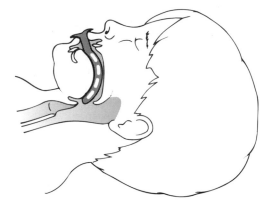

Fig. 9.4 The oropharyngeal airway (Guedel).

presence will stimulate vomiting in a patient who is not deeply unconscious and insertion must be abandoned or the device removed if the patient shows any sign of gagging. The initial upside-down approach avoids pushing the tongue backwards and further obstructing the airway. This is a particular problem in children, but the upside-down and rotate insertion technique is not used as damage may result to the child's teeth or palate. Instead, a tongue depressor is used to depress the tongue, allow the airway to be passed over it to its correct position.

The correct size of airway is one whose length is closest to the distance from the angle of the mouth to the tragus of the ear, or from the centre of the incisors to the angle of the mandible. Generally, a size 2–3 will suit an adult female and a 3–4 an adult male. A larger airway may be needed for very large men.

The nasopharyngeal airway
This is used to enhance an airway in a patient who is not so deeply unconscious, as it tends to be better tolerated than an oropharyngeal device. It is also appropriate in the cases of oral trauma. Select one which is the same diameter as the patient's little finger or generally use a size 6 for a woman and a size 7 for a man. It should be well lubricated and passed via the right nostril (which is usually larger) until the tip lies in the nasopharynx posterior to the tongue. A safety pin through the end of the device will prevent it slipping into the nose and becoming 'lost' in the patient. In a patient lying on their back, the nasal passage runs vertically so the airway must be advanced in this plane and not pointed up towards the patient's cranium. Insertion can cause a little bleeding if it damages the nasal mucosa or a turbinate, so only gentle pressure should be applied to avoid this. The use of this airway is absolutely contraindicated in patients who have a basal skull fracture. The base of the skull is the bony plate, which divides the nasal cavity from the brain. In a head-injured patient it is possible to insert the device into the brain via a fracture of this bony plate.

The pocket mask

The pocket mask is a clear soft plastic facemask with a one-way valve and a port for attaching an oxygen supply. The mask is placed over the patient's nose and mouth and held in place with both of the rescuer's thumbs, the rescuer's index and middle fingers gripping the angle of the mandible.

A head tilt–chin lift manoeuvre can now be applied and the patient ventilated by blowing expired air through the one-way valve. The patient's chest is inspected to ensure it rises as ventilation takes place. Expired gases are vented from the one-way valve away from the rescuer and they are isolated from any vomit or secretions, thus reducing the risk of contamination. Expired air contains 16% oxygen, which will achieve saturations in the patient of about 90%. If oxygen is attached to the mask at flow rate of 10 L/min, the inspired oxygen is raised to 50%, which can bring the patient's oxygen saturation levels to around 98%. Because of the mask's clear construction, any vomit appearing at the patient's mouth can be seen and removed by suction. One size of mask is available, but for paediatric victims, the mask is inverted, the child's chin fitting into the nose part of the mask and the opposite side of the mask lying above the bridge of the nose. It must lie below the eyes to avoid applying pressure to them because this may not only cause damage to the eyes but can also cause vagal stimulation, which can dramatically slow the heart rate.

The bag-valve mask

The bag-valve mask (BVM) device ensures complete isolation from the patient and therefore affords greater protection to the rescuer. The mask

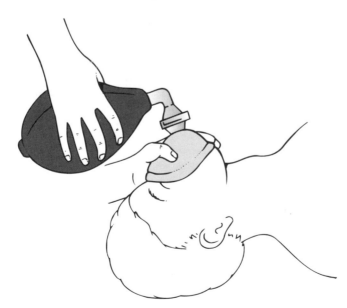

Fig. 9.5 The bag-valve mask (BVM) device.

can be held with one hand, thumb and index finger holding the mask while the middle and ring fingers grip under the mandible and the little finger exerts a jaw thrust behind the angle of the mandible (Fig. 9.5). This leaves the rescuer's other hand free to squeeze the self-inflating bag to ventilate the patient. It is a difficult technique and considerable practice is needed to perform it effectively. The recommended technique for a BVM is for one rescuer to apply the mask with two hands, as described for the pocket mask, and for an assistant, or in some arrest situations for the person doing the chest compressions, to squeeze the bag. Three sizes of bag, designated by bag volume, are available: the 250 mL bag is for neonatal resuscitation only, the 600 mL bag is for infants and small children and the normal, 2000 mL bag is for older children and adults. It is always advisable to use a larger rather than a smaller bag. The victim's chest can be seen to rise and the amount of squeeze adjusted accordingly, whereas if the bag is too small, the patient will be hypoventilated. Using room air, the BVM will deliver 20% oxygen, with oxygen attached at a flow rate of 10–15 L/min (but without a reservoir bag), 50% oxygen is delivered to the patient. The use of a reservoir bag at the same flow rate can bring this to over 90%. The reservoir fills with oxygen during each inspiration of the patient delivering over 90% oxygen to the main bag as it refills during expiration. The oropharyngeal or nasopharyngeal adjuncts can be used with the BVM and the pocket mask but are not a substitute for a good airway position with head tilt–chin lift (or jaw thrust in the patient with suspected cervical spine injury).

The laryngeal mask airway

Having considered ventilation via a mask on the patient's face, the next step moves the mask to the patient's larynx. The laryngeal mask airway (LMA) is a soft rubber mask fitted to a tube. The mask fits over the patient's larynx with its tip lying in the oesophageal opening (Fig. 9.6). The tube houses a standard connector, which allows ventilation devices such as a self-inflating bag and valve to be attached. The LMA is sized from 5 for an adult to 0 for a neonate. In general, larger masks provide better ventilation than smaller ones. The mask is checked for leaks and the tube is inspected for blockage before insertion. The mask is deflated on a flat surface to produce a boat shape. The rescuer stands behind the patient's head while the patient is lying on their back and the LMA is held like a pen, with the index finger between the tube and the point where the inflation tube leaves the cuff.

The tip of the LMA is placed behind the patient's upper incisors and with the index finger holding the tube (Fig. 9.7) it is pushed in the direction of the patient's umbilicus. The LMA is advanced closely applied to the hard and then the soft palates. When the rescuer's finger can go no further into the patient's mouth (Fig. 9.8) the grip is released and the LMA pushed gently home with the other hand holding the end of the tube (Fig. 9.9). The cuff is inflated with the appropriate amount of air, as indicated on the LMA itself. The tube will lift slightly as the cuff is inflated and ventilation with a

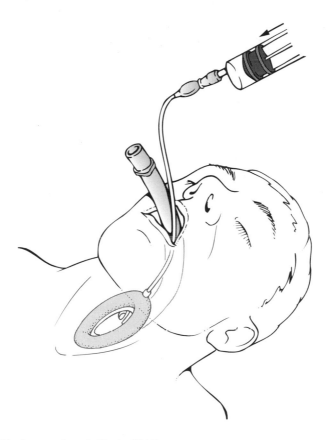

Fig. 9.6 The laryngeal mask airway (LMA).

self-inflating bag attempted. The victim's chest should be seen to rise with inspiration and ventilation is continued. The LMA is not associated with regurgitation and aspiration in unconscious patients who have not previously been ventilated with a BVM.

BVM ventilation can inflate the stomach and cause regurgitation and there is considerable evidence from in-hospital cardiac arrests that primary ventilation by LMA, where licensed users are present, is the optimal method for rapidly and effectively securing a patent airway and ventilating a patient. Evidence from pre-hospital experience of its use in trauma and cardiac arrest is still being gathered but it appears likely that the LMA will be shown to be as effective in pre-hospital airway management. It should be remembered that the LMA is not an alternative to endotracheal intubation, but simply a means of moving the facemask to the larynx: it can be seen as a safe and effective way to ventilate a patient during resuscitation. Although its licensed use is for the resuscitation of unconscious patients, there may be less of a problem using it in a patient who is 'lighter' than

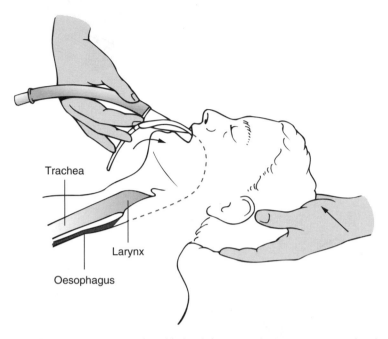

Fig. 9.7 The tip of the LMA is placed behind the patient's upper incisors and with the index finger holding the tube.

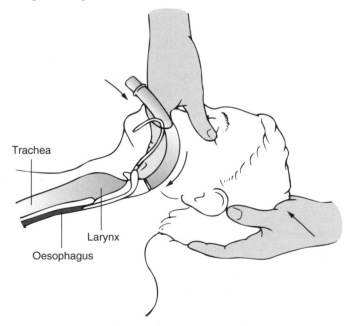

Fig. 9.8 The LMA is advanced closely applied to the hard and then the soft palates.

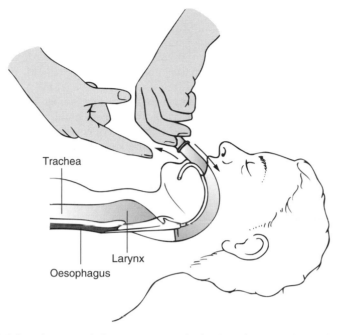

Trachea

Larynx

Oesophagus

Fig. 9.9 When the rescuer's finger can go no further into the patient's mouth the grip is released and the LMA pushed gently home with the other hand holding the end of the tube.

was first thought. The initial stimulation on insertion is of the hard palate, which stimulates a swallowing (suckling) reflex that aids insertion, whereas other techniques stimulate the pharynx, which can cause vomiting. Should vomiting occur with an LMA *in situ*, it should be removed, although the presence of regurgitated material or blood can be managed by gentle suction down the device. If high inflation pressures are required, it is still possible that foreign body obstruction is occurring at the larynx, or that ventilation has caused or aggravated a tension pneumothorax. In this circumstance, the device should be removed and a pneumothorax decompressed, or Heimlich manoeuvres applied or the larynx inspected under direct vision using a laryngoscope as appropriate, depending on the skills of the operator.

Endotracheal intubation
This is the 'gold standard' of airway management. The insertion of a cuffed tube via the mouth into the trachea protects the airway and allows effective ventilation for long periods if required. Although having an endotracheal tube (ETT) *in situ* may be the best way of managing the patient's airway, the process of being intubated is a hypoxic experience and should be completed within 30 s in a patient who has been preoxygenated for at least 1 min, if possible. Endotracheal tubes are sized according to their internal

diameters and have to be cut to a suitable length prior to use. For a man, a size 9 should be cut to 24 cm and for a woman, a size 8 cut to 22 cm. Two smaller sizes than the one selected should always be available in case difficulty is encountered. For children, the right tube size is approximated from the formula (age/4) + 4, but smaller and larger tubes should always be available. For adults and older children, the tubes have an inflatable cuff to seal the larynx. For size 5 tubes and below, the tube is uncuffed, as it will fit more exactly in the near circular cricoid ring of the child (see chapter 11).

The ETT is inserted with the aid of a laryngoscope, which is used to gain a view of the larynx; levering will cause the view to be lost. In an unconscious or anaesthetized patient BVM ventilation with 100% oxygen is performed for at least 1 min before insertion, to saturate fully the patient's haemoglobin. Laryngoscopes, tubes, inflation syringe and connectors are assembled and checked prior to an intubation attempt and high-flow suction must be available.

The laryngoscope is held in the left hand and the tip of its blade inserted into the right of the patient's mouth. As it is inserted, it is moved to the midline sweeping the tongue with it. The handle of the laryngoscope will now be at about 45° to vertical, pointing upwards in the direction of the patient's feet. The handle is lifted along this 45° line, lifting the tongue and the mandible to provide a view of the vocal cords. Lifting the patient's head may help to bring the cords into view. The tube must be seen to pass through the cords before the laryngoscope is removed. The cuff is inflated and a self-inflating bag and valve attached to the tube using a catheter mount. The patient is ventilated and the chest should be seen to rise. Auscultation of the chest is required to confirm air entry at both axillae and at both lung bases. No gurgling should be heard over the stomach. When the correct position of the tube has been confirmed, it is secured with tape and ventilation continued.

The usual laryngoscope blade used in adults is the curved Mackintosh variety while a straight blade is more appropriate for infants and children. The tip of the curved blade sits above the epiglottis, lifting it out of the way, while a straight blade sits below the epiglottis and lifts it directly. Note that that the laryngoscope is a lifting device. Although damage can occur to the teeth, palate, pharynx and larynx, the main complication is failure to intubate. As long as failure is recognized within 30 s and ventilation with a BVM re-established, no harm will come to the patient. However, patients have died because of oesophageal intubation and ventilation, which was not recognized by the rescuer. In the event of any doubt, the tube should be removed and the patient ventilated with a BVM system. An end-tidal CO_2 monitor will detect the presence of carbon dioxide to confirm the correct position of the tube, as well as auscultation. If the tube is in the trachea, CO_2 is detected but is absent if it is lying in the oesophagus. Finally, the chest must always be seen to rise on inspiration.

Endotracheal intubation requires considerable skill and experience. A resuscitation situation is not the right time or place for the inexperienced to practice. If trained but out of practice, the operator may be allowed one

Table 9.1 The percentage of oxygen delivered to the patient by different airway management systems

Method	% O_2 delivered to patient
Expired air ventilation	16%
Pocket mask	
Expired air	16%
Plus oxygen at 10 L/min	50%
BVM	
Room air	20%
Plus oxygen at 10–15 L/min	50%
Plus oxygen at 10–15 L/min, plus reservoir bag	90%
LMA or ETT,	
with ventilation using Waters Circuit	95+%

attempt. If they can visualize the cords and intubate within 30 s, all well and good, but valuable time should not be wasted in vain attempts which risk damage. The tube should be withdrawn and the patient effectively ventilated with a BVM or LMA and self-inflating bag to ensure patient safety.

Cricothyroidotomy

In near-complete airway obstruction, where intubation, LMA or BVM ventilation is impossible owing to trauma, a foreign body or anaphylactic oedema, the patient may be insufflated with oxygen via a needle cricothyroidotomy. The skin and soft tissues of the neck are fixed by the operator's left hand, which secures them on either side of the trachea. The membrane between the cricoid and thyroid cartilages is identified.

Using a 12 G Venflon (manufactured by Ohmeda) or a purpose-made device, the membrane is punctured and the cannula advanced into the tracheal lumen. Free air should be aspirated. The catheter is connected to a high-pressure oxygen source with a jet insufflator, or oxygen tubing is connected using a side-hole cut and the oxygen set to a flow rate of at least 15 L/min. Occluding the side-hole of the tubing or operating the jet insufflator will direct oxygen into the patient's lungs and the chest should be seen to rise. Expiration is passive and depends on the obstruction being sufficiently incomplete to allow gases to escape via the oropharynx. This technique does not allow for true ventilation since carbon dioxide cannot be excreted and the $PaCO_2$ will rise to lethal levels over about 40 min. It will, however, keep the patient oxygenated and alive while trained help is summoned to secure a definitive airway by, for example, surgical tracheostomy. An adaptation of this technique is to pass a seldinger wire through the needle which has penetrated the cricothyroid membrane and to pass it in a retrograde fashion through the vocal cords, to retrieve it through the back of the mouth. An ETT can then be 'railroaded' over the wire into the trachea, the guide wire then being removed as the tip of the tube passes the cricothyroid puncture, thus securing the airway. Complications of cricothyroid puncture include failure, haemorrhage due to puncturing the thyroid blood vessels and surgical emphysema from insufflating a cannula that has been misplaced in the tissues surrounding the trachea.

DECOMPRESSION OF A TENSION PNEUMOTHORAX

Ventilating a patient with a BVM, LMA or ETT can exacerbate a tension pneumothorax in a victim of trauma or in a patient who has received external chest compressions. Tension pneumothorax is a life-threatening condition that must be managed quickly and effectively. It means that the pleural membrane has been punctured and air is entering the pleural space on every inspiration, but a one-way valve has been created which prevents the air from escaping. Gradually, the ever-increasing pneumothorax compresses the affected lung and the rise in pressure causes the collapse of the lung, a mediastinal shift and tracheal deviation towards the opposite side. The pneumothorax must be immediately decompressed with a 14 G Venflon, which punctures the chest wall on the affected side at the second intercostal space in the mid-clavicular line, allowing the air to escape. A hiss of escaping air will confirm the diagnosis and improve ventilation. The needle is removed and the catheter left in place. If a tension pneumothorax had not been present, the catheter is left *in situ* as an iatrogenic pneumothorax might otherwise ensue. As soon as is practicable, a definitive chest drain should be inserted in the fourth intercostal space in the mid-axillary line and connected to a closed system bag or underwater seal.

CONCLUSION

Without an airway we die. It is vital for us all to know and be competent in carrying out the basic manoeuvres of head tilt–chin lift and jaw thrust. They also form part of the more advanced techniques described in this chapter. The two-handed pocket mask and BVM techniques will, together with suction and oxygen, effectively manage nearly all airway and breathing problems. The LMA is a considerable improvement on BVM, yet is simple to learn and apply and reduces the risk of inflating the stomach and causing regurgitation. Endotracheal intubation is the gold standard of airway management but requires a technique demanding considerable skill and experience. There is no merit in attempting and failing a more advanced method and subjecting the patient to the risk of cerebral hypoxia when a simpler technique would achieve effective ventilation and oxygenation of the victim. Points to remember:

- Without a patent airway the patient cannot be ventilated
- Without ventilation, for more than 3–5 min, hypoxic brain damage may occur
- Ventilation must be confirmed by chest movement or by auscultation after intubation with an endotracheal tube or laryngeal mask

- If the correct position of the tube cannot be confirmed, it should be removed and the patient reoxygenated by other means before another attempt is made
- The best method of airway management is that which secures the best ventilation and oxygenation for the patient
- The jaw thrust should be used if cervical spine injury is a possibility
- If cervical spine injury is a possibility, cervical spine control must be simultaneous with airway management.

REFERENCES

Davies P R, Tighe S Q, Greenslade G L, Evans G H 1990 Laryngeal mask airway and tracheal tube insertion by unskilled personnel. Lancet 336(8721):977–979

Stone B J, Leach A B, Alexander C A 1993 The laryngeal mask in cardiopulmonary resuscitation. Resuscitation 65:245–248

Stone B J, Leach A B, Alexander C A et al. 1994 The use of the laryngeal mask airway by nurses during cardiopulmonary resuscitation. Anaesthesia 49:3–7

Stone B J, Chantler P J, Baskett P J F 1998 The incidence of regurgitation during cardiopulmonary resuscitation: a comparison study of bag valve mask v laryngeal mask. Resuscitation 38:3–6

Defibrillation

Ruth Austin   Alison Snow

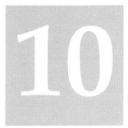

■ CONTENTS

INTRODUCTION

Early defibrillation is undoubtedly a vital link in the chain of survival and is the definitive treatment for ventricular fibrillation (VF) (European Resuscitation Council 1998). The aim of this chapter is to:

- Outline the basic principles of cardiac anatomy and physiology
- Consider the causes of VF and the importance of defibrillation
- Discuss factors that may influence the success of defibrillation
- Present the procedure that should be followed when administering a defibrillatory shock to a patient
- Consider new developments in defibrillation techniques.

BACKGROUND ANATOMY AND PHYSIOLOGY

In order to understand how defibrillation works, aspects of the basic anatomy and physiology of the heart need to be considered. The main mass of the heart (in both atria and ventricles) consists of muscular tissue (the myocardium). The myocardium is made up of specialized involuntary cardiac muscle. Similar to skeletal muscle cells, myocardial cells are made up of actin and myosin (Ganong 1995) and are grouped in bundles within a connective tissue framework, which carries small blood and lymphatic vessels and autonomic nerve fibres (Jowett & Thompson 1989).

The muscle fibres in the myocardium branch and connect with each other, giving the appearance of a sheet of muscle rather than a large number of individual cells. The ends of the cells are in close contact with each adjacent cell, joined by intercalated discs, within which are gap junctions that allow muscle action potentials to spread from one fibre to another (Tortora & Grabowski 1993). This is why as soon as contraction starts in any part, it spreads through the entire network of muscle cells; thus, contraction cannot remain localized. A ring of fibrous tissue separates the atria and ventricles; therefore, when a wave of contraction passes over the atrial muscle it can only spread to the ventricles through the conduction system (Wilson 1987).

The conduction system

All cardiac muscle cells have the intrinsic ability to beat, but there are also certain specialized muscle cells (automatic cells) that make up the conduction system. These cells are able to initiate and conduct electrical impulses within the heart, which in turn produce myocardial contraction (Jowett & Thompson 1989).

The conduction system is made up of several parts (Fig. 10.1). The sinoatrial (SA) node (1) is situated in the right atrium and acts as the primary pacemaker of the heart, because of its intrinsic ability to rapidly generate and conduct impulses. These impulses spread throughout the atrial fibres, down to the atrioventricular (AV) node. The AV node (2) is located in the atrial septum through which the impulse then travels to the bundle of His (3) and then down the right and left bundle branches (4), which are situated through the intraventricular septum. The impulse then travels through the Purkinje fibres (5), which rapidly conduct the impulse into the mass of ventricular muscle (Tortora & Grabowski 1993).

Electrophysiology

Electrolyte concentrations within cardiac cells and in the extra cellular fluid are of major importance for electrical stimulation of the heart. Those involved in a cardiac action potential (changes in voltage across the cell

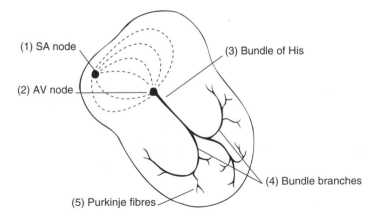

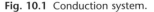

Fig. 10.1 Conduction system.

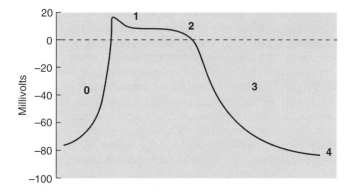

Fig. 10.2 Digram showing the action potential in myocardial cells: 4 = polarization, 0 = depolarization and 1–3 = repolarization. See text.

membrane) are potassium (mainly intracellular), and sodium and calcium (mainly extracellular). There are three separate phases of electrical activity in myocardial cells during the generation of an action potential (Fig. 10.2).

1. *Polarization (phase 4)*. At rest, the myocardial cell has a membrane potential of −90 mV and is said to be polarized.
2. *Depolarization (phase 0)*. When the cell is electrically activated, positively charged sodium and calcium ions flow into the cell. The cell now has a positive charge (while the surrounding extracellular fluid has a negative charge), thus allowing electrical current to flow from cell to cell.
3. *Repolarization (phases 1–3)*. This is the process through which the cell is returned to its resting state by means of the active sodium pump in which potassium, calcium and sodium return to their original sites via channels in the cell membrane. Once a cardiac muscle cell has been depolarized, it takes 200 ms to return to a state in which it can be repolarized again (the absolute refractory period). The refractory period is therefore the time interval when a second contraction cannot be triggered (during depolarization and most of repolarization). This time is necessary to give the ventricles time to fill with blood before contraction (depolarization). It is, however, a 'vulnerable period' because stimulation at this time will sometimes initiate VF.

Ventricular fibrillation

Ventricular fibrillation is chaotic electrical activity within the chambers of the heart, resulting in loss of coordinated myocardial contraction (Bossaert 1997). This chaotic contractile activity of the myocardial muscle cells results in the absence of any pumping action, which stops blood flow and thus oxygen supply to the vital organs, including the heart itself. Unless VF is terminated by defibrillation and blood flow is sustained by basic life support (BLS), myocardial ischaemia, anoxia and acidaemia will occur within 2–3 min and death will result (Inwood & Cull 1997, Resuscitation Council (UK) 1998).

Ventricular fibrillation is usually triggered when an area of ischaemic or infarcted myocardium becomes irritable. Early warning signs of myocardial irritability may be multifocal ventricular ectopics or the R-on-T phenomenon, where an R wave of a premature ventricular complex falls onto the T wave of the preceding beat. This is likely to initiate VF because the T wave represents the repolarization phase when the myocardium is unstable, that is, in its 'vulnerable' period. Increased concentrations of circulating catecholamines (usually because of chest pain), metabolic abnormalities and certain drugs can exacerbate this sensitivity and irritability further. Other causes may be respiratory failure (Resuscitation Council (UK) 1998), electrocution, poisoning, hypothermia or hyperthermia, drowning and some drugs such as tricyclic antidepressants (Flanders 1994, Bossaert 1997), all of which may result in acidosis and hypoxia adversely affecting the myocardium.

Ventricular fibrillation is the most common initial arrhythmia that occurs in sudden cardiac arrest (Skinner & Vincent 1997). Indeed, it has been suggested that 80–90% of adults who collapse because of nontraumatic cardiac arrest are found to be in VF when first attached to a cardiac monitor (Varon et al. 1998).

IMPORTANCE OF DEFIBRILLATION AND SURVIVAL

The use of electrical current on the hearts of mammals has been reported as long ago as 1775 (Driscol et al. 1975), but it was not until 1947 that Claude Beck defibrillated a human heart by using an internal defibrillator (Hermreck 1988). In 1956, Zoll et al. described the successful use of an external defibrillator on a human.

All defibrillators are made up of a power source (mains (ac) and/or rechargeable batteries), which charge a capacitor to a pre-set level, and electrodes through which the stored energy is discharged. The energy delivered is usually measured in joules but success relies on the flow of current, which is measured in amperes (Resuscitation Council (UK) 1998). The purpose of external defibrillation is to deliver an electrical current through the heart which is sufficient to depolarize the critical mass of myocardial cells, thus allowing the natural pacemaking tissues, usually the SA node, to resume control.

Ventricular fibrillation will not self-correct and will therefore persist until death, unless rapid defibrillation is carried out (Flanders 1994). The patient has the best chance of survival, when the time between VF starting and defibrillation occurring is as short as possible. The chances of successful defibrillation occurring decrease at a rate of 7–10%/min (Bossaert et al. 1998). The longer VF persists, the greater the energy requirement for defibrillation. Indeed, the threshold can increase to as much as five times as VF continues (Bossaert 1997).

Since nurses are often first on the scene of a cardiac arrest, it is vital that they can defibrillate in order to maximize the chances of survival. Tunstall-Pedoe et al. (1992) suggest that over 80% of successful defibrillations are achieved within the first three shocks. Cooper & Cade (1997) found that with just the implementation of regular BLS updates for nurses, immediate patient survival increased by 5.2% over a 3-year period. When coronary care nurses were taught to defibrillate, a 72.9% immediate patient survival rate was seen, compared with 43.2% for patients treated by the hospital resuscitation team (Cooper & Cade 1997). However, it must be remembered that survival is heavily influenced by underlying physiological condition and patients in a coronary care unit are more likely to have a prime cardiac arrhythmia than those elsewhere in the hospital.

If defibrillation does not occur, VF will degenerate into asystole after about 15 min. It should be remembered that VF cannot always be successfully defibrillated and the current flowing through the thorax will depend upon a number of factors:

- Transthoracic impedance
- Defibrillation waveforms
- Energy requirements
- Influence of drugs.

Transthoracic impedance

Transthoracic impedance is the amount of resistance between the two defibrillator paddles/electrodes. This resistance affects the flow of electrical current to the heart and is influenced by many factors. It is important that paddle size and position is correct. Adult paddles are 10–13 cm in diameter, with one positioned to the right of the sternum below the clavicle and one at the apex of the heart (V4–V5 position; see Fig. 10.3). Using an anterior posterior paddle position may be useful if refractory VF is experienced; however, in practice, it may be difficult if only hand-held paddles are available. The impedance between the skin and the paddles is reduced by the use of gel pads or electrode paste, which improves conduction. The use of electrode paste may be problematic since it can smear across the chest

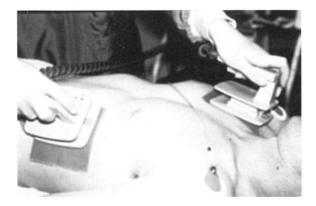

Fig. 10.3 Defibrillator electrode/paddle position during defibrillation (reproduced with permission of Resuscitation Council (UK).

during cardiopulmonary resuscitation (CPR) and this will cause the shocks to arc across the chest (Bossaert 1997). Firm contact with the paddles to the chest will reduce transthoracic impedance and it is recommended that 12 kg of pressure is applied (Bossaert & Koster 1992). Some models of defibrillator have a light on the paddles, which indicates whether adequate contact with the patient's chest wall has been achieved. It is of interest to note that in a recent study Deakin *et al.* (1998b) concluded that there was no significant difference in transthoracic impedance between standard defibrillation paddles and self-adhesive defibrillator pads (the latter do not require 12 kg of pressure). Impedance is generally increased if the lungs are full of air; therefore, timing the shocks with the expiratory phase of ventilation is recommended. Recent research suggests that positive end-expiratory pressure of 20 cm H_2O can increase transthoracic impedance by 6% and is best reduced by disconnecting patients from bagging circuits or ventilators during defibrillation (Deakin *et al.* 1998a).

Defibrillation waveforms

External defibrillators deliver a short but intense electrical current through paddles or adhesive pads (Chapman 1997). However, very little of the electrical energy delivered reaches the myocardium – some research states that it can be as little as little as 4% (Lermann & Deale 1990). The defibrillation waveform is the pattern of this current as it is delivered and is the subject of research since the reaction of the heart varies with different waveforms. Waveforms are influenced by the way they are generated and by transthoracic impedance. At present, there are two commonly used waveforms (Fig. 10.4a and b). The first is a truncated exponential waveform generated by discharging energy stored in a capacitor through the chest and then halting the current abruptly before the discharge is complete. The pattern of the waveform is seen to quickly reach a peak and then to decrease slowly until it drops suddenly back to zero (Fig. 10.4a). The second is a damped sinusoidal waveform in which generated energy is discharged through an inductor to the patient (Fig. 10.4b). This allows the current gradually to reach a rounded peak, which then slowly returns to zero (Bardy *et al.* 1995, Chapman 1997). The peak current attained is considered one of the determining factors of successful defibrillation (Dazell & Adgey 1991, Bossaert & Koster 1992, Chapman 1997).

Each waveform can be grouped according to the number of phases (changes in the direction of current flow) that it is composed of. Current that flows one way between electrodes is monophasic and current that flows in two directions is biphasic (Fig. 10.4c). Since the early 1990s, internal defibrillators have used biphasic waveforms and there are many researchers who believe that using these waveforms for external defibrillation will allow a decrease in the energy requirements (Tang *et al.* 1989, Bardy *et al.* 1995). Research is, however, limited and has mainly been carried out in animal laboratories where VF is induced and only present for a few seconds before defibrillation. Out of the laboratory (either in-hospital or out-of-hospital), VF is often caused by ischaemia and frequently occurs in a hypoxic, acidotic heart with coronary artery disease. Combine this with a heart that has been fibrillating for several minutes and the exact effects of different waveforms on a heart are still not known. Some studies in the USA have investigated the efficacy and clinical benefits of low-energy biphasic defibrillators in out-of-hospital arrests but results are inconclusive. However, members of the European Resuscitation Council have stated that

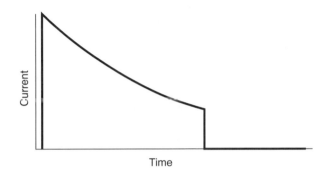

Fig. 10.4 Defibrillation waveforms: (a) Monophasic truncated exponential waveform.

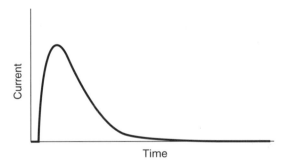

Fig. 10.4b Monophasic damped sinusoidal waveform.

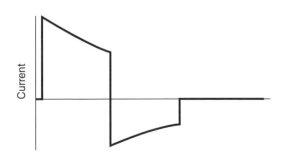

Fig. 10.4c Biphasic truncated exponential waveform.

the use of alternative waveforms is acceptable if they are of the same or greater benefit to patients in VF.

Energy requirements

The energy selected is an important factor – too much could damage the myocardium and too little would be ineffective – and so the energy used is a balance between these risks. The first shock for defibrillating VF is 200 J (American Heart Association 1992, European Resuscitation Council 1998) and because transthoracic impedance is significantly lowered by the first shock, the second is repeated at 200 J. If this fails then the third is increased to 360 J (Varon *et al*. 1998).

Influence of drugs

Oxygen is possibly the most important drug used in cardiac arrest. Hypoxia will compromise the contractility and electrical stability of the myocardium, which in turn decreases the threshold for VF and limits the effects of catecholamines (Skinner & Vincent 1997). Therefore, the highest concentration possible should be given to all patients during resuscitation attempts.

Adrenaline

Adrenaline (epinephrine), a naturally occurring catecholamine, is the next most commonly used drug during cardiac arrest. It is a powerful α and β antagonist with the following effects:

- Peripheral vasoconstriction
- Increase in cerebral and coronary perfusion
- Increase in myocardial contractility.

It is seen as an adjunct to BLS but defibrillation should not be delayed in order to administer it.

Other antiarrhythmics

The use of other drugs during cardiac arrest remains controversial (Bossaert 1997). If refractory VF is present then pharmacological intervention can be considered with drugs such as lignocaine (lidocaine) or bretylium. Both increase the fibrillation threshold, but lignocaine is known to increase the defibrillation threshold and, therefore, energy requirements (Bossaert 1997, Skinner & Vincent 1997; see chapter 7).

PREPARATION OF THE PATIENT

Adequate preparation of the patient for defibrillation is vital in order to achieve the desired outcome. Gel pads should be placed on the patient where the paddles are positioned. They not only help reduce transthoracic impedance, they also protect the patient's skin from being burned. The pads should be changed every three to six shocks because they can quickly dry out, making them less effective (Inwood & Cull 1997). However, manufacturer's guidelines do vary and this is an area of resuscitation under investigation. It should also be remembered that despite the use of gel-pads, burns could still occur, particularly in patients receiving multiple shocks (Pagan-Carlo et al. 1997). The location of the paddles aims to allow the maximum depolarization of the myocardial tissues when the shock is delivered. Bone is a poor conductor of electricity and therefore neither paddle should be placed over the sternum. It has been suggested that the most frequent mistakes made when defibrillating are improper use of gel pads, poor contact with the chest wall and incorrect positioning of paddles (European Resuscitation Council 1998).

SAFETY ISSUES

It is important to remember that while defibrillation is often lifesaving, it can also be potentially harmful. Obviously, for a patient in VF, the risk of skin burns or myocardial muscle damage is worth taking. However, for the person delivering the shock, and other people present, keeping the risks low is paramount. Although rare, injuries to staff of shocks to the hands and legs resulting in burns and tingling sensations have been reported (Gibbs et al. 1990). When defibrillation takes place, it is essential that no part of any person be in direct contact with the casualty. The operator must shout 'Stand Clear!' and perform a visual check that everyone does so before delivering the shock (Resuscitation Council (UK) 1998).

Other safety measures to consider include checking that the chest wall is dried of any blood or body fluid (Inwood & Cull 1997) that may conduct the shock. There are reports that delivering a shock over glyceryl trinitrate patches can cause a small explosion (Moore 1986). Therefore, all transdermal patches or ointments should be removed from the chest wall before defibrillation (Bossaert & Koster 1992).

Oxygen is another potential danger, owing to the risk of ignition by any sparks caused by defibrillation. It is important that paddles are not placed over anything metal, for example jewellery or ECG electrodes and care should be taken to take oxygen masks and bag-valve mask devices away from the patient when defibrillation is carried out.

If the patient has a permanent pacemaker, the defibrillation paddles should be placed at least 12.5 cm away from it (Resuscitation Council (UK) 1998). Most modern pacemakers have a protection circuit fitted, which makes damage from defibrillation unlikely; however, there is a small risk that current may travel down the electrode and cause burns to the endocardium. This may disrupt the pacing threshold and cause loss of capture, so permanent pacemakers should be checked after successful defibrillation (Skinner & Vincent 1997, Resuscitation Council (UK) 1998).

DEFIBRILLATION PROCEDURE

1. Confirm in the patient the absence of cardiac output by performing a 10-s carotid pulse check.

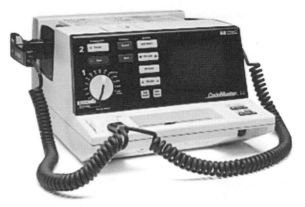

Fig. 10.5 Manual defibrillator (reproduced with permission of Hewlett Packard Ltd, Health Care Group).

2. Attach patient to defibrillator using either gel pads and paddles or monitoring leads to interpret the ECG rhythm (see Fig. 10.5).
3. If rhythm is VF or pulseless ventricular tachycardia (VT), 200 J should be selected (gel pads and paddles should be placed on the chest if not already done).
4. A visual check is performed by the operator to ensure that all staff are clear and a verbal order to 'stand clear' given.
5. The paddles are charged while maintaining firm pressure with the paddles on the patient's chest.
6. The operator checks the monitor to confirm rhythm is still shockable.
7. Discharge the defibrillator by pressing both paddle discharge buttons simultaneously.
8. Keeping the paddles on the patient's chest, the rhythm should be reassessed visually. A pulse check is only necessary if the rhythm has changed to one that is compatible with an output.
9. If VF or pulseless VT is still present a second shock is repeated at 200 J.
10. If a third shock is required, the operator should request that the energy be increased to 360 J.
11. Up to three shocks are delivered in rapid succession (30–45 s), after which if there is no change in rhythm, BLS is commenced and further treatment initiated (see ALS algorithm in chapter 7). Only if there is a delay in charging the paddles between shocks should BLS be carried out until the problem is rectified.
12. Following the three shocks or a rhythm change to a nonshockable rhythm the paddles should be returned immediately to the defibrillator.

SYNCHRONIZED CARDIOVERSION

This is the electrical conversion of atrial and ventricular tachy-arrhythmias that have either not responded to pharmaceutical treatment or are causing haemodynamic compromise. It may be an elective or an emergency procedure. Signs of compromise are chest pain, hypotension, dyspnoea and reduced level of consciousness, all of which would indicate the need for urgent cardioversion. Unlike VF, which is seen as uncoordinated electrical activity, tachy-arrhythmias have identifiable complexes and therefore a vulnerable (refractory) period during the cardiac cycle. It is important that the shock is not delivered randomly because there is a risk of inducing VF. Timing or synchronizing defibrillation to occur on the R wave of the QRS complex reduces this risk. Synchronization is achieved by switching the 'sync' button on (the button is located on the front of most defibrillators). The QRS complexes are detected and the R-wave is usually marked with a dot or an arrow on the monitoring screen. To deliver a shock, preparation of the patient and safety considerations are the same as for manual defibrillation. However, it must be remembered that there may be a short delay from when the discharge buttons are pressed until the energy is delivered to the patient, while the defibrillator detects an R wave. Paddles should therefore remain firmly on the patient's chest until the shock has been delivered.

It is essential that for both planned and emergency cardioversion anaesthetic support is present in order to sedate the patient and safely manage the airway. Defibrillation is unpleasant and painful, therefore synchronized or non-emergency shocks should only be given after the patient has been given analgesia as well as sedation.

AUTOMATIC INTERNAL CARDIOVERTER DEFIBRILLATOR (AICD)

Patients who have AICDs fitted are increasingly being seen in the UK and it is important to know how to deal with them should a patient require defibrillation. AICDs are composed of a pulse generator with one or more sensing electrodes and are used to sense and treat certain arrhythmias. These devices are implanted in patients for whom conventional treatments have failed (James 1997). Modern AICDs are placed in a similar position to permanent pacemakers and are able to carry out anti-tachycardia pacing, low-energy synchronized cardioversion, high-energy defibrillation and pacing for brady-arrhythmias (Causer & Connelly 1998). Fricker (1997) suggests that as many as 200–300 patients are fitted with AICDs each year in the UK. If the AICD fails to work appropriately, the patient may suffer a cardiac arrest and defibrillation should be carried out as though the AICD is a pacemaker.

NEW DEVELOPMENTS

Automatic external defibrillators

Doctors have traditionally carried out defibrillation, as they were believed to be more capable of identifying cardiac rhythms (Mckee *et al.* 1994). However, several studies have demonstrated that many doctors have poor knowledge and skills in the management of ventricular fibrillation (David & Prior-Willeard 1993, Lowenstein *et al*. 1981, Tham *et al*. 1994). Nursing staff are more likely to be present first at cardiac arrests but are often not suitably trained to use a defibrillator, so there may be unnecessary delay before patients are defibrillated, thereby reducing the chances of successful resuscitation. Cummins (1990) states that this is unacceptable in clinical areas where defibrillators are available. Training tends to be targeted at nursing and medical staff working in acute areas where cardiac arrests are expected; however, approximately 50% of in-hospital cardiac arrests occur in nonacute areas (Tunstall-Pedoe *et al*. 1992).

To increase the availability of defibrillation, the advisory external defibrillator (AED) was developed in the early 1970s in America. Its design was originally aimed at personnel who might be involved in pre-hospital arrests such as fire fighters, emergency medical technicians and the general public (Cummins 1989) (see Fig. 10.6a). In recent years, the use of AEDs in hospitals has increased (Mckee *et al*. 1994, Kaye *et al*. 1995, Warwick *et al*. 1995, Destro *et al*. 1996). Its main feature is that rhythm analysis for VF is automatic, creating several advantages:

- Personnel only need to be able to recognize cardiopulmonary arrest, attach the AED to the patient, follow its instructions and carry out BLS
- A lower level of training is required and some centres routinely incorporate AED training into BLS sessions (Kaye *et al*. 1995)
- Shocks can be delivered more rapidly because many machines automatically charge to a pre-set level
- Its simplicity enables a wide range of both medical and nonmedical personnel to use it.
- Safer to use because of 'hands-free' defibrillation by the operator (see Fig. 10.6b).

This type of defibrillator falls into two categories: totally automatic or semi-automatic. Both require that self-adhesive electrodes be attached to the patient's chest in the normal positions. Once turned on, totally automatic defibrillators will automatically charge when VF is detected and deliver a shock. Semi-automatic defibrillators will visually and/or verbally instruct the operator to deliver a shock and may or may not charge automatically. Following a shock, some units will automatically reanalyse and others require the operator to press the analyse button. Most AEDs will analyse within 10–25 s. There is no need to perform pulse checks or BLS between shocks, as this would interfere with the analysis, so contact should not be maintained with the patient during shock sequences. The third shock will automatically go up to 360 J and subsequent shocks will remain at 360 J.

Semi-automatic defibrillators can be overridden and used as manual defibrillators. Many also have facilities for synchronized cardioversion, three-lead ECG and oxygen saturation (SpO_2) monitoring, and external pacing.

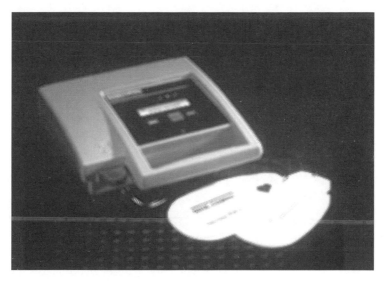

Fig. 10.6a Automatic external defibrillator (reproduced with permission of Physio-Control UK Ltd).

Measured transthoracic impedance

Current-based defibrillation as an alternative to energy-based defibrillation is under investigation. Defibrillators that can measure transthoracic impedance are being developed. By measuring impedance, the exact current necessary is determined and amperes are then selected rather than joules. This means that patients with a high impedance would receive enough current and those with low impedance would not receive too much (Varon *et al.* 1998).

NURSES' RESPONSIBILITIES

Documentation

Following a cardiac arrest, nursing staff must not only clearly document the specific treatment interventions and outcomes in the patient's notes, but also be accountable for any actions or decisions that they made (UKCC 1996). Records should clearly identify the patient's name, date, times and must include a signature of the nurse writing the report. A printout from the defibrillator should be attached into the medical notes, particularly if defibrillation occurred before medical staff were present. There is now more demand to assess the standards and effectiveness of resuscitation attempts and many hospitals audit arrests. If required, nursing staff must complete the appropriate forms for audit or research purposes (see chapter 8).

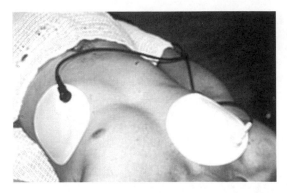

Fig. 10.6b Hands-free defibrillation (reproduced with permission of Resuscitation Council (UK)).

Checking equipment

Following the Kings Fund Audit in 1994 it is recommended that emergency medical equipment should be checked daily. Indeed, defibrillators should be discharged daily according to manufacturer's guidelines. While this may seem ritualistic and mundane, it will enable staff to become familiar with what equipment is available in their particular clinical area. Trained nurses should be carrying out the checks, but it should not be designated to just one or two members of staff.

Training and skills retention

Nurses have both a professional and legal responsibility to maintain the technical skills that are necessary to competently and safely carry out defibrillation. This can be encouraged and supported first by those carrying out training, and second by nursing management to enable release from clinical areas for training. Skills are known to deteriorate rapidly (Wynne *et al*. 1987, Crunden 1991) and some advocate attending update training every 3 months (Flanders 1994, Bossaert 1997). There have been some encouraging results when assessing skills and memory retention following AED training courses (Kaye *et al*. 1995, Mckee *et al*. 1994). Even so, nurses' perception of their own skills is rarely accurate (Kaye & Mancini 1986, Inwood 1996) and, alarmingly, long-serving nurses are less likely to attend training (Crunden 1991).

CONCLUSION

Early defibrillation is a vital link in the chain of survival since it is the single most effective treatment for VF (see Fig. 10.7). The speed at which it occurs has a direct affect on survival.

Defibrillation is a potentially dangerous procedure and must be carried out safely, immediately. While not all nurses are trained to defibrillate, they should understand why it is necessary, how it is done and be able to assist

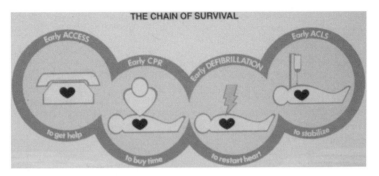

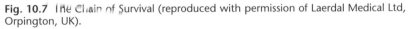

Fig. 10.7 The Chain of Survival (reproduced with permission of Laerdal Medical Ltd, Orpington, UK).

in an emergency. Health care professionals should look towards increasing access to defibrillators. It is likely that 'hands off' defibrillation will improve the safety aspects of the procedure and new developments such as biphasic and current-based defibrillators will change the way in which that it is achieved. Bossaert (1997) believes that defibrillation should be a basic requirement for *all* nurses and perhaps with the advent of AEDs this may become a possibility.

Regardless of what changes scientific research and technology may produce, nurses will continue to be key personnel in carrying out defibrillation in hospital cardiopulmonary resuscitation.

REFERENCES

American Heart Association 1992 Standards and guidelines for cardiopulmonary resuscitation (CPR) and emergency care. Journal of the American Medical Association 268:919–934

Bardy G H, Gliner B E, Kudenchuk P J, Poole J E, Dolack G L, Jones G K, Anderson J, Troutman C, Johnson G 1995 Truncated biphasic pulses for transthoracic defibrillation. Circulation 91(6):1768–1774

Bossaert L 1997 Fibrillation and defibrillation of the heart. British Journal of Anaesthesia 79:203–213

Bossaert L, Koster R 1992 Defibrillation: methods and strategies. Resuscitation 24:211–225

Bossaert L, Handley A, Marsden A, Arntz R, Chamberlain D, Ekstom L, Evans T, Monsieurs K, Robertson C, Steen P 1998 European Resuscitation Council guidelines for the use of external defibrillators by EMS providers and first responders. Resuscitation 37:91–94

Causer J P, Connelly D T 1998 Implantable defibrillators for life threatening ventricular arrhythmias. British Medical Journal 317:762–763

Chapman F 1997 Defibrillation impedence: a current affair. InSync 4(1):20–21

Cummins R 1989 From concept to standard of care? Review of the clinical experience with automated external defibrillators. Annals of Emergency Medicine 18:1269–1275

Cummins R 1990 Encouraging early defibrillation: the American Heart Association and automated external defibrillators. Annals of Emergency Medicine 19:1245–1248

Crunden E 1991 An investigation into why qualified nurses inappropriately describe their own cardiopulmonary resuscitation skills. Journal of Advanced Nursing 16:597–605

Cooper S, Cade J 1997 Predicting survival, In-hospital cardiac arrests: resuscitation variables and training effectiveness. Resuscitation 35:17–22

David J, Prior-Willeard P F S 1993 Resuscitation skills of MRCP candidates. British Medical Journal 306:1578–1579

Dazell G W, Adgey A A 1991 Determinants of successful transthoracic defibrillation and outcome in ventricular fibrillation. British Heart Journal 65:311–316

Deakin C D, McLaren R M, Petley G W, Clewlow F, Dalrymple-Hay M J R 1998a Effects of positive end-expiratory pressure on transthoracic impedence – implications for defibrillation. Resuscitation 37:9–12

Deakin C D, McLaren R M, Petley G W, Clewlow F, Dalrymple-Hay M J R 1998b A comparison of transthoracic impedance using standard defibrillation paddles and self-adhesive defibrillation pads. Resuscitation 39:43–46

Destro A, Marzaloni M, Sermasi S, Rossi F 1996 Automatic external defibrillators in the hospital as well? Resuscitation 31:39–44

Driscol T E, Ratnoff O D, Nygaard O F 1975 The remarkable doctor Abildgaard and counter-shock. Annals of Internal Medicine 83(6):878–882

European Resuscitation Council–Advanced Life Support Working Group 1998 The 1998 European Resuscitation Council guidelines for advanced life support. British Medical Journal 316:1863–1869

Flanders A 1994 A detailed explanation of defibrillation. Nursing Times 90(18):37–39

Fricker J 1997 Clinicians count the cost of implantable defibrillators. Lancet 349:105

Ganong W F 1995 Review of Medical Physiology, 1st edn. Prentice-Hall, Englewood Cliffs

Gibbs W, Eisenberg M, Damon S 1990 Dangers of defibrillation: injuries to emergency personnel during patient resuscitation. American Journal of Emergency Medicine 8(2):101–104

Hermreck A S 1988 The history of cardiopulmonary resuscitation. American Journal of Surgery 156:430–436

Inwood H 1996 Knowledge of resuscitation. Intensive and Critical Nursing Care 12: 33–39

Inwood H, Cull C 1997 Defibrillation. Professional Nurse 13(3):165–168

James J E 1997 Living on the edge – patients with an automatic internal cardioverter defibrillator (AICD): implications for nursing practice. Nursing in Critical Care 2(4):163–168

Jowett N J, Thompson D R 1989 Comprehensive coronary care, 1st edn. Scutari Press, Harrow, pp. 14–35

Kaye W, Mancini M E 1986 Retention of cardiopulmonary resuscitation skills by physicians, registered nurses, and the general public. critical care Medicine 14(7):620–622

Kaye W, Mancini M E, Giuliano K K, Richards N, Nagid D, Marler C, Sawyer-Silva S 1995 Strengthening the in-hospital chain of survival with rapid defibrillation by first responders using AEDs: training and retention issues. Annals of Emergency Medicine 25(2):163–168

Kings Fund 1994 Organisational Report. Kings Fund, London

Lermann B B, Deale O C 1990 Relation between transcardiac and transthoracic current during defibrillation in humans. Circulation Research 67:1420–1426

Lowenstein S R, Hansborough J F, Hill D, Mountain R, Scoggin C, Libby L S 1981 Cardiopulmonary resuscitation by medical and surgical house officers. Lancet ii:679–681

Mckee D R, Wynne G, Evans T R 1994 Student nurses can defibrillate within 90 seconds. Resuscitation 27:35–37

Moore S 1986 Jump starting the heart. Journal of Emergency Nursing 12(4):213–217

Pagan-Carlo L A, Stone M, Verber R E 1997 Nature and determinants of skin 'burns' after transthoracic cardioversion. The American Journal of Cardiology 79(5):689–691

Resuscitation Council (UK) 1998 Advanced Life Support course provider manual, 3rd edn. Resuscitation Council (UK), London

Skinner D V, Vincent R 1997 Cardiopulmonary resuscitation, 2nd edn. Oxford University Press, Oxford

Tang A S, Yabe S, Wharton J M, Dolker M, Smith W M, Ideker R E 1989 Ventricular defibrillation using biphasic waveforms: the importance of phasic duration. Journal of American College of Cardiology 14:207–214

Tham K Y, Evans R J, Rubython E J, Kinniard T D 1994 Management of ventricular fibrillation by doctors in cardiac arrest teams. British Medical Journal 309:1408–1409

Tortora G J, Grabowski S R 1993 Principles of anatomy and physiology, 7th edn. Harper Collins, New York, pp. 591–623

Tunstall-Pedoe H, Bailey L, Chamberlain D, Marston A, Ward M, Ziderman D 1992 Survey of 3765 cardiopulmonary resuscitations in British hospitals (the BRESUS Study). British Medical Journal 304:1347–1351

UKCC 1996 Guidelines for professional practice. UKCC, London

Varon J, Marik P E, Fromm Jr R E 1998 Cardiopulmonary resuscitation: a review for clinicians. Resuscitation 36(2):133–145

Warwick J P, Mackie K, Spencer I 1995 Towards early defibrillation – a nurse training programme in the use of utomated external defibrillators. Resuscitation 30:231–235

Wilson K J W 1987 Anatomy and physiology in health and illness, 6th edn. Churchill Livingstone, Edinburgh, pp. 61–97

Wynne G, Marteau T, Johnston M, Evans T, Whiteley C 1987 Inability of trained nurses to perform basic life support. British Medical Journal 294:1198–1199

Zoll P M, Linenthal A J, Gibson W, Paul M H, Norman L R 1956 Termination of ventricular fibrillation in man by externally applied countershock. New England Journal of Medicine 254:727–732

FURTHER READING

Quinn T 1998 Cardiopulmonary resuscitation: new European guidelines. British Journal of Nursing 7(8):1070–1077

Paediatric resuscitation

Caz Holmes

INTRODUCTION

The resuscitation of a child, whether of a neonate or a 12-year-old, is always stressful for everyone involved. The death of a child seems to go against the normal pattern of life and it is unrealistically expected that every person will live their allotted three-score years and ten. Sadly, children do die but unlike adult deaths, very few paediatric deaths are expected and managed. Even in children who are known to have life-limiting conditions, their deaths commonly occur following an acute episode and are therefore sudden and unplanned. Although there has been remarkable development in providing palliative and terminal care, it still appears that professionals find it difficult to withhold resuscitation attempts in children, especially when an acute episode precipitates cardiac arrest.

This chapter does not aim to discuss the ethics of withdrawing or withholding of treatment in children but rather focuses on the following :

- The pathways of paediatric arrests
- The possible prevention of paediatric arrests
- The procedures of paediatric resuscitation
- The problems often encountered in paediatric arrests
- The pains often experienced in paediatric arrests.

Reflective practice should be actively engaged in as part of all nurses' professional development. It should not be feared, or thought to be a pointless exercise, since by asking only three simple questions nurses can enhance their learning from experience by determining why the event went well or otherwise. Nurses at all levels of experience should ask after any critical incident (not only after a resuscitation event):

- What did it feel like, how was it for me?
- What went well and what would I want to emulate next time?
- What would I want to be different or do differently next time?

These questions are discussed in more detail later in the chapter.

PATHWAYS OF PAEDIATRIC CARDIAC ARREST

One of the most important differences between adult and paediatric arrests is the precipitating cause of arrest. Children rarely have cardiac arrests caused by myocardial infarction as they do not have underlying coronary heart disease. There are two major conditions that are likely to precede cardiac arrest in children: hypoxia and circulatory failure.

Hypoxia

In childhood, most cardiac arrests are secondary to hypoxia (American Heart Association 1997, Advanced Life Support Group 1997). This may be due to respiratory failure, with precipitating factors being infection such as bronchiolitis, asthma, epiglottitis and birth asphyxia. Prior to the child having respiratory failure from these causes, they will exhibit many signs of respiratory distress.

Respiratory arrest may also be a result of neurological dysfunction caused by certain poisons or during prolonged fitting, raised intracranial pressure caused by either a head injury or secondary to space-occupying lesions. These result in respiratory depression which eventually leads to respiratory arrest; however, it is important to realize that severe neuronal damage will have occurred before the respiratory arrest. If appropriate intervention does not occur, then a full cardiopulmonary arrest is precipitated. In these situations, the preceding respiratory distress may not be identified. Whatever the cause of the respiratory arrest, by the time cardiac arrest occurs the child has already had a period of respiratory insufficiency that will have caused hypoxia and respiratory acidosis. The combination of hypoxia and acidosis causes cell damage and cell death, particularly in more sensitive organs such as the brain, liver and kidney, but before myocardial damage is severe enough to cause cardiac arrest.

Circulatory failure

The other cause of cardiac arrest in children is secondary to circulatory failure (American Heart Association 1997). More commonly called 'shock', circulatory failure occurs because of fluid loss (e.g. from haemorrhage, gastroenteritis or burns) causing hypovolaemic shock or from fluid maldistribution caused by sepsis, anaphylaxis and heart failure. All organs become deprived of essential nutrients and oxygen as shock progresses, and cardiac arrest will follow since circulatory failure, like respiratory fail-

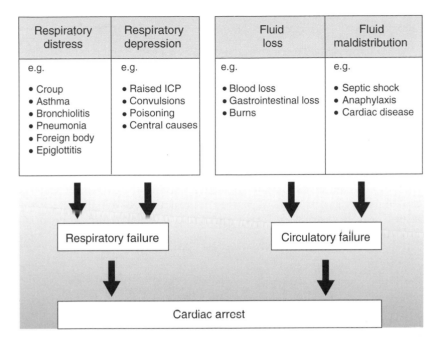

Respiratory distress	Respiratory depression	Fluid loss	Fluid maldistribution
e.g.	e.g.	e.g.	e.g.
• Croup • Asthma • Bronchiolitis • Pneumonia • Foreign body • Epiglottitis	• Raised ICP • Convulsions • Poisoning • Central causes	• Blood loss • Gastrointestinal loss • Burns	• Septic shock • Anaphylaxis • Cardiac disease

Respiratory failure   Circulatory failure

Cardiac arrest

Fig. 11.1 Pathways leading to cardiac arrest in childhood (with examples of underlying causes) (Advanced Life Support Group, 1997, with permission of BMJ Publishing Group).

ure, causes tissue hypoxia and acidosis. The pathways leading to cardiac arrest in children are shown in Figure 11.1.

With regard to the outcome of paediatric resuscitation, the worst outcome is for children who have suffered an out-of-hospital arrest and who arrive at hospital apnoeic and pulseless (American Heart Association 1997, Advanced Life Support Group 1997). These children have a poor chance of complete neurological survival since there has often been a prolonged period of hypoxia and ischaemia before the start of adequate cardiopulmonary resuscitation. Early recognition of seriously ill children is vital to prevent respiratory and/or cardiac arrest and provision of paediatric cardiopulmonary resuscitation training for the public could improve the outcome for these children.

It is vital for health-care professionals looking after children to be able to assess the child and recognize potential respiratory and/or circulatory failure. All respiratory distress has the potential to develop into respiratory failure and all shock has the potential to develop into circulatory failure. Nurses are very good at carrying out frequent observations on their patients, sometimes every 10–15 min in some cases. However, many nurses are poor at interpreting the observations and putting them into context (see Box 11.1).

Box 11.1 Preventing respiratory and/or cardiac arrest in children

The key to preventing respiratory and/or cardiac arrest in children is
• a structured assessment
• correct interpretation of the assessment
• delivering the appropriate intervention.

As with all resuscitation training, the ABC, (Airway, Breathing, Circulation) approach is imperative in both basic life support (BLS) and advanced life support (ALS) and should be seen as part of an on-going cycle of constant re-evaluation. A child's condition can rapidly deteriorate unnecessarily if there is failure to reassess continually, since this failure will lead to a delay in providing the vital and appropriate intervention.

The important message to communicate in resuscitation training is

1. To assess using the ABC approach,
2. To act accordingly and then
3. Immediately reassess, act accordingly and then reassess.

This must continue until the situation has been stabilized or considered futile and so discontinued.

POSSIBLE PREVENTION OF A PAEDIATRIC ARREST

In contrast to the adult, the sick child gives many indications that they are deteriorating. Moreover, it is crucial that health-care providers are able to assess and interpret these signs. Accurate assessment and interpretation of the findings should then result in appropriate intervention, thus preventing a cardiac arrest occurring. The key to being able to prevent a cardiac arrest is to be able to diagnose that the child is in respiratory and/or circulatory failure. The term *diagnosis* is often thought to be of the domain of only medical staff. However, since it is generally the nursing staff that perform regular observations on the child, they have a professional (as well as moral) duty to be able to interpret these observations and determine whether the child is manifesting respiratory and/or circulatory insufficiency. If the nurse concludes that the child is in such a compromised condition and the need for urgent treatment is recognized, medical assistance can be summoned and treatment initiated to prevent the child deteriorating to the point of cardiac arrest. It is the prevention of this state that will increase the likelihood of survival and reduce morbidity. It is important to remember a child can rapidly progress to asystole, but only after a period of tachycardia and then bradycardia. It is the skill of recognizing respiratory and/or circulatory insufficiency that all nurses and doctors who care for children need to acquire.

RAPID CARDIOPULMONARY ASSESSMENT OF THE INFANT OR CHILD

This assessment uses the ABC approach used in cardiopulmonary resuscitation (CPR).

A. Airway patency
• Able to maintain independently – indicated by crying, talking, or obvious shifting of air
• Able to be maintained with assistance – indicated by improved shifting of air/reduction of stridor, grunting, etc., with airway opening manoeuvres or use of airway adjuncts
• Unmaintainable – indicated by inability to shift air and requiring interventions such as intubation, removal of foreign body or cricothyroidotomy.

B. Breathing
• Rate – concern if rapid, slow or absent
• Mechanics – concern if recession/use of accessory muscles, grunting, nasal flaring noted
• Efficiency – concern if inadequate/asymmetrical chest expansion, paradoxical chest movement, presence of breath sounds (crackles or rales on auscultation), stridor or wheeze
• Colour – rather subjective, but hypoxia produces vasoconstriction and skin pallor. N.B. cyanosis is a late and pre-terminal sign of hypoxia. By the time that central cyanosis is visible in acute respiratory disease the child is close to respiratory arrest. In the anaemic child cyanosis may never be visible, despite profound hypoxia. Cyanosis may be present due to cyanotic heart disease, which will be largely unchanged by oxygen therapy.

C. Circulation
• Heart rate – concern if fast, slow (i.e. below 60 beats/min) or absent
• Skin perfusion – concern if capillary refill time is longer than 2 s (but consider ambient temperature)
• Central pulses – concern if weak
• Peripheral pulses – concern if absent
• Colour – rather subjective, but concern if mottled, cold and pale
• Blood pressure – can be a helpful measurement, but note that hypotension is a late and pre-terminal sign of circulatory failure. A child can still be in circulatory failure and have an apparently normal blood pressure. Once a child's blood pressure has fallen, cardiac arrest is imminent. Blood pressure does not diagnose shock but distinguishes between compensated and decompensated shock
• Temperature – concern if a temperature gradient is obvious between central and periphery, with coldness progressing more centrally as circulatory failure progresses. N.B. the temperature gradient can be felt with the hands, with accurate measurements made by a thermometer only when possible

• Central nervous system perfusion – concern if patient is not alert, does not respond to voice or pain, does not recognize parents, is hypotonic. The most important pupillary signs to seek are dilatation, unreactivity and inequality.

This whole assessment should take less than 1 min and should result in the nurse being able to state if the child is in respiratory failure, and/or compensated or decompensated circulatory failure. Failure of either or both systems demands immediate intervention to prevent imminent cardiac arrest occurring.

Note that oxygen should be the first intervention to initiate, while ensuring that medical assistance is on the way.

When any medical intervention is initiated, re-assessment should occur in the same order, i.e. repeat the rapid ABC assessment to establish if there has been improvement or if any further treatment is indicated.

Potential respiratory failure

Rapid cardiopulmonary assessment may result in the nurse concluding that the child's nursing diagnosis is potential, rather than actual respiratory failure or shock. Frequent and sequential assessments must continue and oxygen administration instigated in a non-threatening manner whenever possible. Infants should be supported with their head in the neutral position and older children allowed to assume a position of maximum comfort to minimize the work of breathing and to optimize airway patency.

Actual respiratory failure

If signs of actual respiratory failure are present, a patent airway must be established and adequate ventilation ensured with maximum supplemental oxygen provided. When signs of shock are present, vascular access should be established rapidly and volume and medications administered as needed.

When cardiopulmonary failure is detected, initial priority is given to ventilation and oxygenation. If circulation and perfusion fail to improve rapidly, treatment for shock should be given. If, however, cardiopulmonary arrest occurs, cardiopulmonary resuscitation must be commenced.

THE PROCEDURES OF PAEDIATRIC RESUSCITATION

Paediatric basic life support

Paediatric BLS is not simply a scaled-down version of that given to adults. Although the general principles are the same, specific techniques are required in order to give the optimum support to the child. The techniques used vary according to the child's age. Current guidelines (Bossaert 1998) split children into three age bands: the infant being any child under the age of 12 months, a young child being between the ages of 1 and 8 years, and an older child being greater than 8 years of age. These age bands are somewhat artificial, and, if effective cardiopulmonary support is not being achieved, then the technique should be changed accordingly. BLS is vital in the child. Since the largest cause of cardiopulmonary arrest is hypoxia, oxygen delivery is the critical requirement in children (rather than the need for defibrillation as in adults), and prompt access to ALS is also required.

The sequence of BLS for children is similar to that for adults. The sequence begins by initially establishing that the environment is safe to approach, ensuring that the rescuer does not become a second victim. Responsiveness should be established by gentle shaking and talking to the child, looking for facial response such as crying, grimacing and eye opening. The gentle shaking should be performed on the torso of the child and never involve the head and neck because of the risk of causing cerebral bleeding. Children showing signs of respiratory distress, but still managing to breathe for themselves, will often position themselves to maintain patency of a partly obstructed airway. They should be allowed to remain in the position that is most comfortable for them. Once unresponsiveness has been determined the single rescuer should shout for help but stay with the child in order to provide BLS, if necessary, for approximately 1 min before going and getting help. Airway-opening manoeuvres should follow finding an unconscious child since relaxation of muscles and passive posterior displacement of the tongue may lead to airway obstruction; therefore, whenever an unconscious, non-breathing victim is found, the airway should be opened immediately. This is usually accomplished by the head tilt–chin lift manoeuvre (see also chapters 6 and 9). The head is tilted to the neutral position in the infant (ear in line with the shoulder) and the sniffing position in the child (tilting the head a little further than the neutral position, but avoiding the over-extension of the neck that is achieved in adult resuscitation). If neck injury is suspected, head tilt should be avoided and the airway opened by a jaw thrust (see chapter 9) while the cervical spine is completely immobilized.

Once the airway is opened, the rescuer must determine whether the child is breathing. The rescuer looks for a rise and fall of the chest and abdomen, listens for exhaled air and feels for exhaled airflow on their cheek. If spontaneous breathing is present, a patent airway must be maintained. If the infant or child is unresponsive, has no evidence of trauma and is obviously breathing effectively the rescuer should place the child in the recovery position. If no spontaneous breathing is detected then rescue breathing must be commenced ensuring that the patent airway is maintained by a head tilt–chin lift or jaw thrust. Five rescue breaths should be administered creating visible chest rise.

Rescue breaths are the most important support for the non-breathing infant or child, where the rescuer covers the infant's nose and mouth with their mouth, or pinches the nose and covers the mouth only in the child greater than 1 year. There is wide variation in the size of paediatric victims so it is impossible to make precise recommendations about optimal pressure or volume of ventilations. The volume and pressure should be sufficient to cause the chest to rise. If the child's chest does not rise during rescue breathing, ventilation is not effective. If air does not enter freely, either the airway is obstructed or more breath volume or pressure is necessary. Improper opening of the airway is the most common cause of airway obstruction and the rescuer should be prepared to re-attempt opening the airway and re-attempt ventilation if initial ventilation attempts are unsuccessful. If rescue breathing fails to produce chest rise after four re-attempts to open the airway, a foreign-body airway obstruction must be suspected and the rescuer should proceed to the Removal Of Foreign-Body Algorithm (see Fig. 11.2).

Once rescue breaths have been successfully achieved, only then should the rescuer proceed to assessing the circulation. A pulse should be felt for up to 10 s, locating the brachial pulse in the infant (half-way between the elbow and shoulder pushing firmly against the humerus) and the carotid pulse in a child greater than 1 year. If the rescuer can feel a heart beat at a rate of one, or more than one beat per second (i.e. greater than 60 beats/min) then cardiac massage is not required. The child is in a state of respiratory arrest, therefore support of the respiratory system is vital: single rescue breaths should be given at a rate of approximately 20/min – i.e. one breath every 2–3 s. If the rescuer discovers the heart rate to be slower than one beat per second (i.e. less than 60 beats/min) the child's heart is in bradycardia which could rapidly progress to asystole. Cardiac massage should be commenced immediately, using the correct age-specific landmarks (Box 11.2).

Box 11.2 Age-specific landmarks

In the infant, the area of compression is found by imagining a line between the nipples and compressing over the sternum one finger-breadth below this line. Two fingers are used to compress the chest to one-third of the chest's depth. There is an alternative method often favoured in the neonate where infant cardiac compression can be achieved using the hand-encircling technique: the infant is held with both the rescuer's hands encircling the chest. The thumbs are placed one finger-breadth below the imaginary inter-nipple line and compression carried out. This method is limited by the size of the infant versus the size of the rescuer's hands and care must be taken so as not to squeeze fingers and thumbs towards each other, ensuring compression by thumbs only.

In the child, the lower margin of the child's rib cage is identified on the side of the chest nearest the rescuer, locating the notch where the ribs and the sternum meet (the xiphisternum). It is important that compressions are not done over the xiphisternum. The long axis of the heel of one hand is placed over the long axis of the lower half of the sternum (between the nipple line and the xiphisternum). The fingers of the hand should be lifted to ensure that pressure is not applied to the child's ribs. The chest is compressed to approximately one-third of the chest depth. In children over the age of approximately 8 years, it may be necessary to use the 'adult' two-handed method of chest compression to achieve the adequate depth of compression.

Once the correct age-specific landmarks have been made, the chest should be compressed at a rate of about 100 times a minute (a little less than two compressions a second). After five compressions, tilt the head, lift the chin and give one effective ventilation as before. Return your fingers or hand immediately to the correct position on the sternum and give a further five compressions and continue.

The infant and child should be reassessed after 20 cycles of compressions and ventilations (approximately 1 min) for any resumption of spontaneous breathing or pulse. Continue with further chest compressions and ventilations as needed, reassessing every 20 cycles. If the rescuer is still on their own after the first 20 cycles and no one has responded to the shout for help then the rescuer must the contact the emergency services. An infant can be taken to the telephone by the rescuer but if the child is too large to comfortably carry (and run with), they should be left while the emergency phone call is made, and returned to in order to re-establish BLS. Resuscitation should be continued in the 5:1 compression–ventilation ratio until

- The infant or child shows signs of recovery
- Advanced life support is able to be initiated by the emergency services, or
- the rescuer becomes exhausted.

The cardiopulmonary resuscitation manoeuvres recommended for infants and children are summarized in Table 11.1.

Removal of foreign body algorithm

If difficulty in achieving effective breathing is experienced, despite attempts to reposition the airway and ensuring a chin lift, then foreign body airway obstruction sequences should be followed. A number of deaths from foreign body aspiration occur in the preschool-age child and virtually anything may have been inhaled. The diagnosis is rarely clear-cut, but should be suspected if the onset of respiratory compromise is sudden. It is vital to note that airway obstruction may also occur with infections such as acute epiglottitis and croup. In such cases, attempts to relieve the obstruction using the methods described below are dangerous.

Children with known or suspected infectious causes of airway obstruction, and those still breathing and in whom the cause of obstruction is unclear should be taken to hospital urgently. The physical methods of clearing the airway, described below, should therefore only be performed if:

- The diagnosis of foreign body aspiration is clear-cut and dyspnoea is increasing or apnoea has occurred
- Head tilt/chin lift and jaw thrust has failed to open the airway of an apnoeic child.

If the infant (or child) is breathing spontaneously, its own efforts to clear the obstruction should be encouraged. Intervention is necessary only if these attempts are clearly ineffective and breathing is inadequate. Blind

Table 11.1 Summary of basic life support techniques for different ages

	Infant (up to 1 year)	Younger child (approx. 1–8 years)	Older child (over approx. 8 years)
Airway opening manoeuvres	Head tilt–chin lift to the neutral position. Use jaw thrust if trauma suspected	Head tilt–chin lift to the sniffing position. Use jaw thrust if trauma suspected	Head tilt–chin lift to the sniffing position. Use jaw thrust if trauma suspected
Breathing	Five rescue breaths, sealing over nose and mouth	Five rescue breaths, pinching nose and sealing over mouth	Five rescue breaths, pinching nose and sealing over mouth
Circulation assessment	Brachial pulse	Carotid pulse	Carotid pulse
Compression technique	Two fingers on sternum, one finger breadth below inter-nipple line, or encircle chest and place thumbs as for fingers	Heel of one hand on lower sternum avoiding xiphisternum	Two interlocking hands with heel of lower hand on lower sternum, avoiding xiphisternum
Compression rate	Approximately 100/min	Approximately 100/min	Approximately 100/min
Compression depth	Approximately 1/3 the depth of the chest	Approximately 1/3 the depth of the chest	Approximately 1/3 the depth of the chest
Compression : ventilation ratio	5 : 1	5 : 1	5 : 1 ideally, or 15 : 2
Cycles per minute	20	20	20 or 6 (if 15 : 2 ratio used)

Box 11.3 Back-blows

- Hold the infant or small child in a prone position and try to position the head lower than the chest.
- Deliver up to five back-blows between the shoulder blades, which creates a sharp increase in pressure within the chest cavity, rather like an artificial cough.
- If this fails to dislodge the foreign body, the rescuer should perform chest thrusts: turn the child to the supine position and give five chest thrusts to the sternum.
- The technique for chest thrusts is similar to that of chest compressions but they are sharper and carried out at a slower rate of 20/min (instead of 100/min), i.e. one every 3 s.

sweeps of the mouth or upper airway should not be performed as this may further impact the foreign body or cause soft tissue damage. If the child is attempting to cough, some assistance may be given by administering back-blows (Box 11.3) coordinated with their coughing – no back-blows should be given when the child is attempting inspiration.

After five back-blows and five chest thrusts the mouth is checked and any visible foreign bodies removed. Reposition the airway by the head tilt/chin lift (jaw thrust) manoeuvre and reassess breathing. If the child is breathing, turn the child on their side and check for continued breathing. If the child is not breathing, administer up to five rescue breaths, attempting to make the chest rise and fall. The child may be apnoeic or the airway only partially cleared. In either case, the rescuer may be able to achieve

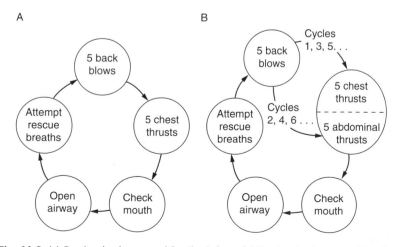

Fig. 11.2 (a) Foreign body removal for the infant. (b) Foreign body removal for the child over 1 year old.

effective ventilation at this stage. If the airway is still obstructed, the sequence of five back-blows then five chest thrusts is repeated for the child under 1 year old. For the child over 1 year old repeat five back-blows but then substitute the five chest thrusts for five abdominal thrusts. Abdominal thrusts are delivered as five sharp thrusts directed upwards towards the diaphragm. Use the upright position if the child is conscious. Unconscious children should be laid supine and the heel of one hand placed in the middle of the upper abdomen. Alternate chest thrusts and abdominal thrusts in subsequent cycles. Repeat the cycles until the airway is cleared or the child breathes spontaneously. Do not use abdominal thrusts in the infant, use five back-blows and five chest thrusts only. Figure 11.2 summarizes the manoeuvres for the removal of foreign body obstruction.

Paediatric advanced life support

If BLS is initiated promptly and performed according to the guidelines, adequate ventilation and circulation may be obtained to reverse the underlying cause of the arrest. It is therefore a 'holding operation', although, on occasions, particularly if the primary pathology is respiratory failure, it may itself reverse the cause and allow full recovery. Failure of the circulation for 3–4 min will lead to irreversible cerebral damage. Delay, even within that time, will lessen the eventual chances of a successful outcome. Emphasis must therefore be placed on rapid institution of BLS and ALS summoned and given as soon as possible.

The paediatric ALS algorithm is, as a model, essentially the same as that for the adult. The biggest difference is that the predominant pathway of arrest in the child will follow the non-ventricular fibrillation (VF)/ventricular tachycardia (VT) pathway (i.e. the right hand side of the algorithm; Fig. 11.3). It is very rare that a child presents in ventricular fibrillation and, therefore, defibrillation is rarely required. However, if it is required, personnel need the knowledge of how to administer the shock. In terms of safety, these are identical to when delivering a shock to an adult but in terms of the shock dose it is extremely different and is discussed later in the text.

The non-VF/VT pathway essentially manifests itself in asystole, extreme bradycardia (i.e. heart rate below 60 beats/min) or pulseless electrical activity (PEA). As can be seen from the algorithm the treatment is not complicated: it requires continued cardiopulmonary resuscitation and adrenaline. What makes the paediatric arrest significantly different from the adult arrest is that there are no easy-grab pre-filled syringes of adrenaline (epinephrine) to give any child. Children are always treated pharmacologically according to their weight, so it is vital in the arrest situation to calculate a working weight. If the child is an inpatient then a recent accurate weight is normally known following the admission procedure. However, if the child's weight is unknown then an estimated weight should be calculated.

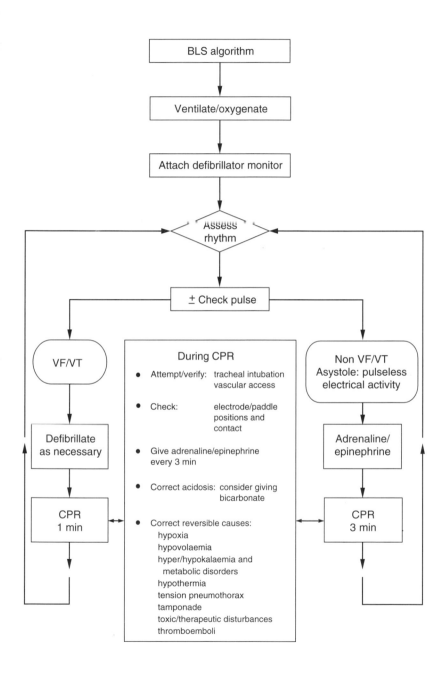

Fig. 11.3 Paediatric advanced life support algorithm (after Resuscitation Council (UK) 1998, with permission).

Box 11.4 Estimated weights

If the child is between 1 and 8 years of age
  Estimated weight (kg) = (age + 4) × 2
  e.g. a 6-year-old's estimated weight = (6 + 4) × 2 = 20 kg
If the child is between 9 and 16 years of age
  Estimated weight (kg) = age × 3
  e.g. a 10-year-old's estimated weight = 10 × 3 = 30 kg

If the age of the child is known then one of the formulae in Box 11.4 should be used.

Alternatively, there are various charts and devices available that enable an approximation of weight to be derived from the child's age, such as the Oakley chart and the Broselow tape, which relates weight to height. This may be particularly useful in accident and emergency (A&E) departments when the child's age may not be known.

As previously discussed it is essential that all nurses caring for children, whether frequently or infrequently, in whatever specialty, should be trained to recognize the signs and symptoms of severe illness which is likely to progress to respiratory and/or circulatory failure if appropriate intervention is not initiated. Within paediatrics, the emphasis is upon prevention of the arrest situation, rather than trying to rescue the child in a cardiopulmonary arrest. A child becomes progressively unwell, sometimes alarmingly quickly, but cardiac arrest in children is not sudden and unexpected, as is often the case in adults, and so these warning signs should be recognized.

Cardiac arrest is typically the result of deterioration in respiratory failure or shock. The terminal rhythm is typically bradycardia with progression to electromechanical dissociation (EMD) also known as PEA or asystole.

The management of the child in arrest will be discussed first. BLS must be initiated immediately and 100% oxygen administered at a high flow rate (15 L/min) as soon as possible. This will normally be given using a bag-valve mask device, remembering that it is essential to use appropriate-sized equipment for the age of the child. The paediatric crash team should be summoned at the earliest opportunity. The child should be monitored as soon as possible, but a pulse check must be done and CPR commenced when it is discovered that the child has no pulse or a rate less than 60/min. The monitor should be used to confirm rather than diagnose the absence of adequate cardiac output.

Asystole, severe bradycardia and PEA require administration of adrenaline as soon as possible and so an administration route needs to be secured. There are three choices:

- Intravenous (IV) access
- Endotracheal (ET) access
- Intraosseous (IO) access.

Box 11.5 Example calculations of adrenaline doses

A 6-year-old in systole *with* IV or IO access
Estimated weight = (6 + 4) × 2 = 20 kg
Adrenaline required = 20 kg × 10 µg/kg = 200 µg
or 20 kg × 0.1 mL/kg = 2 mL of 1:10 000 solution

A 6-year-old in systole *without* IV or IO access
Estimated weight = (6 + 4) × 2 = 20 kg
Adrenaline required = 20 kg × 100 µg/kg = 2000 µg
or, 20 kg × 1.0 mL/kg = 20 mL of 1:10 000 solution
or, 20 kg × 0.1 mL/kg = 2 mL of 1:1000 solution via ET tube

Intravenous access is difficult in the collapsed child, although an experienced paediatrician may be successful. However, if the time taken to find access exceeds 90 s then an intraosseous needle should be inserted if the child has not yet been intubated. Intubation should occur as soon as skilled personnel are available to perform this task. If IV or IO access has been established, adrenaline at 10 µg/kg (0.1 mL/kg of a 1:10 000 solution) should be given (see Box 11.5).

If IV or IO access has not been established but the child has been intubated then adrenaline can be administered via the ET tube, the dosage being 100 µg/kg (i.e. 1 mL/kg of 1:10 000 solution or 0.1 mL/kg of 1:1000 solution; see Box 11.5).

Once adrenaline has been administered, CPR should be continued for 1 min before assessing if output has been restored. The appropriate pulse check should then be made, taking no longer than 10 s to assess whether an adequate output has been achieved. Note that cardiac massage should be suspended when carrying out a pulse check but oxygenation should continue. If the cardiac output is still absent or inadequate, CPR should be restarted and further pulse checks performed intermittently. Further doses of adrenaline should be administered if there is still no output after 3 min. If a second dose of adrenaline is required, the dose should now be given at 100 µg/kg (1 mL/kg of 1:10 000 solution or 0.1 mL/kg of 1:1000 solution). (This is the same calculation as for the first dose of adrenaline given down the ET tube, see above.)

If IV or IO access has still not been secured then the ET tube dose is repeated: ensure that the child never receives more than 100 µg/kg. CPR should then continue, assessing for output intermittently with subsequent doses of adrenaline at 100 µg/kg given every 3 min.

In a prolonged resuscitation, the use of other medications should be considered and underlying reversible causes of arrest should be treated appropriately. Other resuscitation substances that should be considered are listed in Table 11.2.

If the child remains pulseless but an organized complex is visible on the monitor, then they are said to be in a state of PEA, formally referred to as EMD, which can have a number of causes. Outcome after PEA is poor unless the specific cause can be promptly identified and treated. The algo-

Table 11.2 Other resuscitation substances that should be considered

Substance	Indication	Concentration	Dose
IV fluid	Circulatory failure	0.9% normal saline	20 mL/kg
Glucose	Blood sugar < 4 mmol/L	10% glucose	5 mL/kg
Sodium	pH < 7.1 with normal	8.4 % or	1 mmol Eq/kg
bicarbonate	pCO_2 or prolonged arrest and blood gas analysis unavailable	4.2% in neonate	= 1 mL/kg

rithm of chest compressions, hyperventilation using 100% oxygen, intubation and administration of adrenaline should be followed while the cause of PEA is sought. The causes of PEA are:

- Hypoxia
- Hypovolaemia
- Hyper/hypokalaemia
- Hypothermia
- Tamponade
- Tension pneumothorax
- Thromboemboli
- Toxic/therapeutic disturbances.

Ventricular fibrillation

On rare occasions, a child may present in VF. This may be seen in those recovering from hypothermia, those poisoned by tricyclic antidepressants and those with electrolyte imbalance or cardiac disease. It is likely that the child has been found to be pulseless and CPR commenced. VF cannot be diagnosed by a pulse check, only by visual identification on a monitor. VF is a chaotic, disorganized series of depolarizations that result in a quivering myocardium without organized contraction. Ventricular systole does not occur, therefore pulses are not palpable. Resuscitation outcome appears to be considerably better if VF rather than asystole or PEA is the underlying rhythm on initial presentation.

Once VF has been identified as the underlying rhythm, then the child should be quickly prepared to receive defibrillation as soon as possible. CPR can continue until the team is ready to defibrillate. The sequence followed to defibrillate VF is as follows:

1. Continue ventilation with 100% oxygen and chest compressions without interruption, except during defibrillation
2. Apply defibrillation pads to the child, ensuring they do not touch. Classical positioning should be used, i.e. just below the right clavicle and at the left anterior axillary line. For infants, these positions can still be used if paediatric paddles are available, otherwise if only adult paddles are available then apply them to the front and back of the infant's chest

3. Turn on the defibrillator power – the synchronous mode should *not* be selected
4. Select the energy dose – 2 J/kg
5. Stop chest compressions and place paddles in the proper positions on the child's chest
6. Re-check rhythm on the monitor and charge paddles if still in VF
7. All personnel should be told to stand clear and oxygenation discontinued
8. Visually check that no personnel are in contact with the child or bed
9. Firm pressure is applied to the paddles, VF re-confirmed and warning given that a shock is about to be given. Discharge buttons pressed simultaneously
10. ECG evaluated. If VF persists, defibrillator is recharged to same dose (2 J/kg) and personnel warned to stand clear; visually check that no-one is in contact with child or bed, warning given that shock is about to be given then press discharge buttons
11. ECG evaluated. If VF persists defibrillator recharged to third dose (4 J/kg) and personnel warned to stand clear; visually check that no-one is in contact with child or bed, warning given that shock is about to be given then press discharge buttons. Paddles are then placed back into monitor and CPR re-commenced.

Box 11.6 Example calculations

A 6-year-old child in VF, intubated with IV or IO access:
Estimated weight = (6 + 4) × 2 = 20 kg

Defibrillation dose:
  1st dose at 2 J/kg, give 40 J
  2nd dose at 2 J/kg, give 40 J
  3rd dose at 4 J/kg, give 80 J
Adrenaline required:
  20 kg × 10 µg/kg = 200 µg
  or, 20 kg × 0.1 mL/kg = 2 mL of 1:10 000 solution
  Continue CPR for 1 min
If VF persists defibrillate:
  4th dose at 4 J/kg, give 80 J
  5th dose at 4 J/kg, give 80 J
  6th dose at 4 J/kg, give 80 J
Adrenaline required:
  20 kg × 100 µg/kg = 2000 µg
  or 20 kg × 1.0 mL/kg = 20 mL of 1:10 000 solution
  or 20 kg × 0.1 mL/kg = 2 mL of 1:1000 solution
  or continue CPR for 1 min

N.B. No more than 4 J/kg is given. Continue with defibrillation and adrenaline cycles.

If VF persists, adrenaline should be administered at 10 µg/kg (0.1 mL/kg of 1:10 000 solution) and CPR given for 1 min. If VF persists, the heart should be defibrillated with three further shocks at 4 J/kg, followed by more adrenaline 100 µg/kg (1 mL/kg of 1:10 000 solution or 0.1 mL/kg of 1:1000 solution) and 1 min of CPR (see Box 11.6). Repeat the cycle of defibrillation and 1 min CPR until defibrillation has been achieved. Consider the use of other medications and treat reversible causes.

Note that accuracy of joule dosage may be difficult when using defibrillators with stepped energy levels.

PROBLEMS OFTEN ENCOUNTERED IN PAEDIATRIC RESUSCITATION

The most frequent problems that occur during paediatric arrest are:

- Panic
- Problem identifying the team leader
- Petrified of the mathematics
- Presence of parents
- Prolonged resuscitations
- Premonition ignored!

Ways in which these problems can be minimized are discussed below.

Panic

Panic, to one degree or another, is often evident at an arrest (and not only at paediatric arrests). The key to resuscitation attempts running smoothly is to control panic. It seems that paediatric arrests are feared most, both in dedicated paediatric areas and in shared adult and paediatric areas. When it does happen it can often be the start of one's own worst nightmares. This could be due to the fact that paediatric arrests are infrequent and thus many staff have had limited experience of these events. They therefore feel out of their depth, begin to panic, forget what they are supposed to do and in what order. The cardiorespiratory arrest of a child should provoke the immediate calling of the paediatric crash team. Once other people begin to arrive on the scene, effective teamwork can then begin. Delay in getting the right help will only result in increased panic.

1. All personnel should know what the emergency call bell sounds like and how to activate it. It is vital that this is tested on a regular basis. All too frequently someone tries to raise the alarm by activating the emergency call bell only to find no-one comes to their aid because the system has failed, or because staff hadn't realized what the bell signified. There is no excuse for this. It is the first and most vital step in getting help to an arrested child and will then initiate the cascade of getting expert help to the scene as well as equipment. Failure at this stage will cause or increase panic and make the resuscitation attempt less effective.

2. It is essential that every member of the health care team knows how to alert the paediatric crash team in their setting: i.e. what number to call and what to say. All bank and agency staff should be told at the beginning of their shift, as should all locum doctors and other temporary staff.

3. All staff should know where the emergency trolley and equipment are kept so that any one of the staff can get it and take it to the appropriate area quickly.

4. All health care professionals who treat children in their area should be familiar with the paediatric arrest protocols. Education gives knowledge, and knowledge gives enough confidence to keep the panic under control. Lack of knowledge increases the panic and delays appropriate intervention.

Each nursing professional has a duty to 'Safeguard . . . patients, justify public trust, and uphold the good standing and reputation of the profession' (UKCC 1992).

■ **REFLECTION POINT 11.1**   REFLECTION ON ACTION

A new-born female infant failed to respond to the normal sequence of stimulation given at birth and so there was a need for the neonatal crash team to be summoned. The midwife coordinating the delivery requested help from a colleague, asking her to put out a crash call.

She duly ran to the telephone, dialled the correct number, but in her panic did not give adequate information to the switchboard operator. When her call was answered she could only manage to say, 'Quick, quick, quick' and then put the phone down. The operator knew that the call had come from the labour ward and so requested two crash teams to respond – the neonatal and the adult cardiac arrest teams.

This obviously resulted in a myriad of people arriving causing stress to the midwife as the first people to arrive were not from the neonatal team. Eventually, the appropriate people assembled and the extra personnel dispersed, and the resuscitation was successful, although the mother went through enormous stress.

After the incident a debriefing was held, allowing the midwives to talk over how they felt the situation had gone. Both stated that the confusion could have been avoided. When asked how, the first said she could have given her colleague a more directive statement such as, 'Please call 2222 and state neonatal arrest on labour ward.' The second midwife was distraught at her own panic and failing. On being asked what might be done to prevent it happening again, she suggested that rather than just the crash call number being by the phone, a statement of what should be said could be printed, laminated and mounted next to the phone. This suggestion was approved by the midwifery team and thus initiated.

The composition of the paediatric arrest team can itself cause problems. All hospitals have designated personnel who should respond to the paediatric arrest call. This is usually a senior paediatrician, a senior anaesthetist, a resuscitation officer and possibly a senior nurse, as well as the staff already with the arrested child. Sometimes too many people can be in attendance, which can result in confusion as to who is doing what and this can delay appropriate interventions. Equally unsatisfactory is when the expected personnel do not arrive, for one reason or another (e.g. failure of their crash bleep to receive the call). This can delay the appropriate interventions being given. While waiting for the crash team to arrive there are vital steps that the nurse should be instigating. The crash trolley and equipment should be obtained and oxygenating equipment connected. If airway-opening manoeuvres reveal an absence of breathing, artificial ventilation of the child must commence. If there is a delay in getting oxygenating equipment to the child then BLS should be commenced using mouth to mouth/nose resuscitation. Circulation should be assessed and if the heart rate is less than 60 beats/min, cardiac massage must be initiated. There is no excuse for this not being in progress when the crash team arrives. ECG monitoring of the child should also be instigated as soon as possible (see Reflection point 11.1).

Problem in identifying the team leader

Many cardiac arrest situations have been mismanaged because no one person was designated to direct the resuscitation attempt. The team leader role is vital since it ensures a systematic approach to assessment and treatment; it is essential that someone is appointed to this role, or makes it clear that they are appointing themselves to this role. The most suitable person is one who has undertaken paediatric ALS training (they can therefore equally be a doctor, nurse, resuscitation officer or paramedic). Once the team leader has assessed ABC for themselves and ensured that effective ventilation and compressions are being achieved, they should stand back to get an overall view, and direct the resuscitation attempt (e.g. request IV/IO access, request adrenaline, request a pause in compressions to reassess for an output etc. as necessary. The team leader should not become involved in performing tasks.

Nurses give up their role in a resuscitation attempt too easily when doctors arrive and often step aside. However, there is no need for a doctor to take over ventilating the child if the nurse is achieving adequate chest inflation. This is equally true with chest compressions. It makes more sense for nurses to continue with these tasks and let doctors acquire IV access and direct the team. If nurses do not learn to assert their capabilities, they will continue to fear the arrest situation and fail to develop their skills in its management.

All those attending a paediatric arrest will be stressed, no matter how many previous arrests they have attended, and people automatically try to do what they feel most familiar with. For example, when the anaesthetist arrives it is assumed that they will manage the airway. Intubation is not always essential in paediatric arrest and, if a nurse is adequately oxygenat-

---

■ **REFLECTION POINT 11.2** REFLECTION ON ACTION

Following a cardiopulmonary arrest of a 6-month-old infant on a paediatric ward, which resulted in a successful outcome, a debriefing was held for those involved.

The staff nurse who had been performing the massage said, 'I got confused – one doctor said, "stop the massage," and the other said, "continue with the massage," at the same time. I just kept looking from one to the other and didn't know what to do. It was awful not knowing who was right or who I should listen to.'

From further discussion it became evident that there was no clear team leader and that the two doctors present were both asking for things and requesting things to happen. This should not be the case and each doctor should respect their colleagues' knowledge, and be prepared to be led sometimes and not always lead.

The confusion about the massage occurred because the doctors were assessing the output in different places. One was feeling for a femoral pulse and one for a brachial pulse. No femoral pulse was felt and so continuation of massage was requested, whereas a brachial pulse was palpated and so cessation of massage was requested. In the child under one year, output is assessed using the brachial pulse and so the staff were reminded of the paediatric ALS guidelines and the importance of one of the team taking on the role of team leader in a more assertive way. The resuscitation attempt would be smoother and confusion avoided since directives should come from one person.

---

ing the child, it would be better team management for the nurse to continue oxygenation while the anaesthetist acquires IV access, which is another of their expert skills.

If at any one time too many people are in the area and confusion results, the team leader must send some away so that efficiency is maximized (see Reflection point 11.2).

Petrified of the mathematics

One of the commonest fears that nurses have is that they will have to do drug calculations on the spot, in their heads, while everyone is waiting and watching, dreading that they will miscalculate or be unable to control their trembling hands. Unfortunately, there are always calculations to do in a paediatric arrest but it really doesn't have to be a subject of dread. Nurses can overcome this by familiarizing themselves with the charts that are available for estimating weight or ensuring that the formula for estimating weight is visible on the crash trolley. Once the child's weight has been calculated this should be recorded so that it is not recalculated repeatedly. The other calculations are the adrenaline (0.1 mL/kg) and fluids (20 mL/kg). Nurses can practise simulated arrest situations so that they get used to making these quick and easy calculations. Most hospitals insist that ALS skills are updated at least every year and, with the help of resuscitation training officers, simulated situations are an excellent way of putting all theoretical knowledge into practise. It is vital that nurses ensure their own competence by keeping themselves updated in the practice of resuscitation.

Presence of parents

Staff (both nursing and medical) can often feel intimidated if the child's family is present at the arrest. Some parents will realize what has happened and once CPR has commenced will run out from the immediate area, not wanting to witness what happens or fearing that they will be in the way thus preventing their child getting the attention they need (see Reflection point 11.3). Other parents will insist on staying and demand to know what is going on, and why certain things are being done; some may lose control,

---

■ **REFLECTION POINT 11.3** REFLECTION ON ACTION (PRESENCE OF PARENTS)

'I arrived on the ward and was directed to the cubicle where the arrest had occurred. All I could hear was someone screeching at the top of their voice, "Oh my God, Oh my God" – they just didn't stop. Alarms were sounding; a child was in a cot but I could see only his legs. No one was actively resuscitating the child: a nurse was holding a self-inflating bag attached to the oxygen and another nurse was holding a tracheostomy tube; a doctor was being elbowed back by an extremely large lady, who one presumed was the mother. She grabbed the tracheostomy tube from the nurse, still screaming repetitively. It did not appear that anyone was taking control and so, rightly or wrongly, I marched into the room and said in a loud and authoritative voice, "Mrs X, please would you stand out of the way and let us save your child's life!" It sounded very dramatic but it was effective because she became quiet and looked at me. The doctor was then able to approach the child, change the tracheostomy tube and re-establish ventilation.

'I was unable to persuade the mother to leave the cubicle but I continued to talk in a very loud, authoritative voice – rather like giving a running commentary. I was not involved in the arrest "hands on", but I felt that my presence had calmed the situation and that it was no longer a threat. I had never been to an arrest like that before, where a parent actively prevented professionals approaching the child. However, once the mother's hysteria had stopped her presence in the resuscitation room was no longer a problem.'

become hysterical and almost prevent access to their child as they cannot believe or accept that their child is so close to death. This all begs the question, should relatives be allowed in the resuscitation room? Different clinical areas may have different views. For example, it is standard in many A&E departments to exclude family members from the resuscitation room. The rationales being

- That family members do not understand all that goes on during a resuscitation and could regard interventions as cruel
- That family members may hinder the process because if the experience is too traumatic for them they may need attention themselves, creating further confusion
- That it is difficult to 'draw the line' on the number of family who should be present
- That the family may feel you did not try hard enough or long enough or, equally, went on for too long
- That the family might think that nurses and doctors are uncaring in their attitude or think that inappropriate comments were made.

However, most professionals feel it is crucial that the family should be kept fully informed and reassured during the resuscitation (Connors 1996). Recent studies have shown that witnessing resuscitation attempts can be

---

■ **REFLECTION POINT 11.4** REFLECTIONS OF A PARENT

'I had been watching the monitor and things seemed stable, but suddenly the Sister said, "Can I have some help here please – we're losing output." Immediately, a doctor and two staff nurses ran over. One took my child off the ventilator and took over the breathing and one was pumping her chest.

'It was a very odd experience, all so calm and controlled; it felt like I was watching an episode of "Casualty". Another nurse came up to us and said, "It appears Charlotte's heart is not working very well and we need to help her. We are giving her drugs and heart massage. We hope that this will make her heart work efficiently again. You can stay where you are if you want to stay and I'll try and tell you all that happens."

'Then I heard the doctor say, "Stop massage" and I thought Charlotte must be dead. I glanced up and everyone was looking at the monitor. I looked at Charlotte, she looked so small and so dead; she had gone through so much, surely she couldn't die. In fact the monitor showed that her heart had started again and everyone seemed to slip back to doing what they were doing before.

'We saw tremendous teamwork that saved our daughter's life – we will always be grateful.'

helpful for bereaved relatives (Robson 1998; see also chapter 5) although there is a paucity of studies relating predominantly to parents witnessing their own child's resuscitation. Paediatric nurses and paediatricians have the philosophy that the child should not be separated from their parents and family, who should have access to the child in hospital 24 h a day. Therefore, the resuscitation attempt should not be an exception. The caveat to this can only be if the child will not benefit from the family's presence. For example, if the team leader feels that the parents are causing too much distraction and hindering effective resuscitation then this cannot be to the child's benefit; asking the family to leave might be the only option. However, relatives should not be asked to leave as a matter of course and, ideally, someone should be allocated to be with the parents, explaining what is happening and supporting them while they witness events, rather than them just being told that everything possible is being done. The more this happens the more comfortable staff will feel when relatives choose to witness the resuscitation. Should we really deny a family possibly the last moments of their child's life? This is a good topic for discussion among colleagues, especially if real situations that have been experienced are used (see chapter 5; Reflection point 11.4).

Prolonged resuscitations

Some resuscitation attempts can cause great anxiety particularly to nursing staff, when the resuscitation is prolonged. In hospital, it is the responsibility of a senior paediatrician to make the decision when to stop resuscitation. However, this is easier said than done because the natural drive of wanting to save a child's life can override objectivity (see Reflection point 11.5).

Paediatric resuscitation often used to be prolonged, with every possible drug being drawn up and administered despite their inappropriateness. Since the implementation of agreed algorithms, fewer attempts with all the anti-arrhythmic drugs occur. If there has been no detectable signs of cardiac output, and there has been no evidence of cerebral activity despite up to 30 min of cardiopulmonary resuscitation it may be reasonable to stop resuscitation. The duration of the resuscitation attempt should not be the major factor in the decision whether to continue. Exceptions to this rule include:

■ **REFLECTION POINT 11.5**   REFLECTIONS ON PRACTICE

'He was brought into A&E, navy blue, cold and rigid. The ambulance crew had to start CPR when they picked the child up and so we had to continue and gave ALS. It seemed wrong and unnecessary – he was so obviously dead. Why can't ambulance crew be allowed to certify someone dead? It's hard to give it your all in a situation you know to be futile – so why even start it? The memory is haunting and upsetting.'

- The hypothermic child – resuscitation must continue until the core temperature is at least 32 °C or cannot be raised despite active measures
- Children who have taken an overdose of cerebral depressant drugs such as phenobarbitone

In these cases, prolonged resuscitation attempts will be necessary. There is increasing concern that litigation could arise if a resuscitation attempt leaves a child with permanent brain damage. Nevertheless, the decision to terminate resuscitation efforts must be based solely on cardiovascular unresponsiveness in the presence of effective oxygenation and ALS.

Premonition ignored

Nurses can experience immense frustration and anxiety when the concerns they have expressed to the medical team about the condition of the child are ignored. There are, unfortunately, stories told of arrests that have occurred that might have been prevented. Nurses may inform the medical team a number of times about their concern for the child, either from accurate interpretation of a child's observations or from intuition (recognized and described by Benner 1984) conceived out of a wealth of experience in children's nursing. A less experienced doctor may delay appropriate intervention instructing only further observation, but later have to respond to a cardiac arrest call for the very same child (see Reflection point 11.6). The

---

■ **REFLECTION POINT 11.6**   REFLECTIONS ON ACTION

'Her blood pressure was dropping, she was tachycardic and her CVP was 8. I informed the doctor and an albumin bolus was prescribed at 10 mL/kg. This made no difference to the blood pressure, CVP was 10 and she remained tachycardic. I felt uneasy and informed the doctor that I was concerned. Another fluid bolus was prescribed but I did say that I didn't think she was underfilled. However, further fluid was given but little change occurred as a result except her CVP was 20.

'She was opening up a temperature gap and was looking grey. I informed the Sister in charge about my concerns and she went to speak to the doctor who came back to me and jokingly said, "Pestering me again?" I said that I was concerned because there had been no response to the volume and that she just wasn't right. I asked if there could be a chance of cardiac tamponade but was told it was unlikely and that maybe we should restart her inotrope. Her gases were going off and I was sure something sinister was going on so I took a deep breath and went and found the consultant. He immediately came and assessed the patient and requested an echocardiogram. Her BP suddenly fell and she became bradycardic, although massage was not initiated. The echo revealed a considerable cardiac tamponade and cardiocentesis was performed under echo control: 120 mL of blood was aspirated!

- Why didn't the doctor listen to me earlier?
- Why wasn't the doctor as concerned as me?
- What else could I have said or done?

'I felt guilty for not being more vocal but pleased that I had spoken to the consultant directly. In a strange way I was pleased that I had been right in my diagnosis and that I was proved right to have concerns. This experience has given me greater belief in my own abilities.'

result may be that nurses may feel angry that their warnings were not heeded; they may feel guilty that they were not vocal enough and should have taken their concerns to a more senior level and therefore feel that the arrest was somehow their fault. The doctor may feel guilty for not recognizing how sick the child was, despite warnings from nursing staff. This may then lead to feelings of incompetence or lack of confidence, which results in failure to lead the arrest in an effective way. Parents may be angry. that no one did anything earlier.

In a situation like this, people are often looking to apportion blame, which can result in poor teamwork, unresolved questions and can foster bad working relationships. In this type of situation, whatever the outcome of the resuscitation, discussion with the relevant personnel is vital, so that lessons can be learned from the experience. If the resuscitation attempt proved unsuccessful then facilitation of the group discussion is beneficial from someone who was not involved and who can be objective. When there has been a conflict of beliefs then support must be made available for all levels involved. Structured reflection upon this kind of experience is crucial if nurses want to move on rather than allowing a bad experience to inhibit their development, damage their self-confidence and threaten their trust in their colleagues. They must answer the following questions:

- What happened?
- Why did it happen?
- What did I do?
- How did I feel?
- What would I do differently next time?

There are a number of structured reflection models available for use, for example Johns' (1993) Model. Parents will want to ask many of the same questions and have the right to do so. This can cause extra stress for all those involved and may evoke even more feelings in the nurse that might also need to be worked through using structured reflection.

THE PAINS IN PAEDIATRIC RESUSCITATION

The death of a child is one of the most tragic events that anyone can experience and can leave staff, as well as parents and other family members, stunned by their inability to have prevented the child's death. Most paediatric deaths are sudden and unexpected, with few child deaths being managed in the way adult death can be. Nurses in A&E departments are often presented with a child who is brought in apnoeic and pulseless. Resuscitation attempts, although known to be futile, are normally initiated but rarely prolonged. Since ambulance crew have to initiate BLS on finding a victim unresponsive, apnoeic and pulseless, ALS has to be given in order to be sure that the child was given every chance of recovery. Sudden infant death syndrome (SIDS) is a parent's worst nightmare, especially as no explanation can be given for the cause of the death. The law requires that the child's death be fully investigated, which means the police are involved and the child has to undergo a post mortem. This causes additional pain and stress to the family, and nursing staff can feel very awkward in this situation. They have empathy with the devastated family yet appreciate the need for an investigation. A nurse may feel a conflict of interest and might find the experience very emotional.

All nurses know that they will at have to face death and dying at some point in their career, but if the first death they experience is that of a child many will find it particularly difficult. Infant mortality rates in the western world are relatively low and few experience the death of a child. Life expectancy has increased over the years and younger parents often have not experienced death of a relative before. It is even more devastating if your first experience of bereavement is the loss of your own child.

The resuscitation attempt and death of a child are very difficult to cope with emotionally, but nurses have the additional pain of caring for the grieving parents. Nurses will help them to perform last offices, take a photograph and a handprint of the child and finally leave the hospital without their child, knowing that they must return to their home where the child's toys and belongings wait for them in silence; this causes a great sense of grief to nursing staff. It is usually a nurse who accompanies the parents and family to the mortuary when they return the following day to once again see their child. The pain of not knowing what to say can cause considerable mental turmoil and heartache.

Another situation that can be painful for nurses is when the child is thought to have died from a non-accidental injury. The nurse has to remember that they are there to nurse the child and family and not to act as judge and jury. Injury may have been caused deliberately but the grief the family feels must not be presumed to be any less. This can be a very difficult situation for many nurses and much support may be needed to help that nurse deliver the nursing care expected of them. Structured support should be available afterwards, especially for inexperienced nurses.

The question most frequently asked by family, friends and professionals after the death of a child is, why did this have to happen? There is often no satisfactory answer, although some may find reason through their own faith or beliefs. It is important to remember that individuals have differing beliefs and where one may be comforted by the thought that the child's death is God's will, to another that explanation will be illogical and induce an angry reaction. Events involving a hit-and-run or a drunk driver, or a non-accidental injury or drowning, resulting in death by trauma, generate high stress levels. The pain is very raw and the thought that the child suffered pain and fear prior to death causes much heartache to all involved, whether a member of the family or of the professional services. Staff in areas such as A&E may question why the resuscitation of a 60-year-old alcoholic of no known address was successful but that of the 2-year-old was unsuccessful. Unfortunately, these questions cannot be answered and we have to accept the randomness and inevitability of death. Sadly, it is normal for death to occur at all ages.

Another painful and stressful situation is when a resuscitation attempt has been unsuccessful, but nursing staff are unable to be emotionally involved with the parents and family. This is normally because the situation is perceived in a different way; for example, the child may have severe congenital abnormalities resulting in the child being totally dependent on the parents. The nurse may see the death as 'a blessing in disguise', whereas the parents feel that life has now lost its meaning because the centre of their life has been snatched from them. Nurses who find themselves in a situation where their emotions are disparate from those of the family may have difficulty showing tangible empathy, which can result in the nurse feeling that they have nothing to offer these parents. This results in a relationship that is tense and strained. It is possible that nurses may then begin to feel guilty and angry with themselves, which results in even more barriers to effective communication.

There may be times in paediatric resuscitation that a nurse may feel totally out of their depth and does not know what to do or say. Although there is no substitute for experience, once again education is paramount. It is essential that subjects such as caring for the dying child and their family are put onto the ward's teaching programme, with input from child bereavement specialists or counsellors or from nurses more exposed to such situations. Recommendations for good practice do exist and there is a wealth of literature available on this subject. However, emotions and pain are not something that always fit into a neat formula and once again structured reflection can help the nurse work through their feelings by expressing what happened and why, and exploring whether anything could have been handled differently.

Not knowing what to do or say results in a loss of confidence, which if not explored and resolved will result in low morale, lack of motivation and poor staff retention. Similar situations will be feared and therefore avoided. Although such situations are painful, we can learn to cope, we can learn how to deal with devastated parents and we learn how to support other members of the care-giving team. These tragic situations can be sensitively and confidently managed to allow the family to express their grief in a supportive environment and to guide them through an experience that they do not know how to handle. They will be forever grateful to nursing staff who assisted in the last moments of their child's life. It can be emotionally draining and painful for nursing staff but, at the same time, we know that the pain of death is part of the experience of nursing (see chapter 4). It is our role and our reward to be able to offer comfort and to know that everything possible was done to ensure that the parents do not have any regrets about how they spent their last few hours with their child.

CONCLUSION

I have shown that although sometimes a child's death is inevitable, at other times it may have been preventable. All nursing staff caring for children in their clinical area must have the knowledge and skills to

- Recognize the pathways leading to cardiopulmonary arrest in children
- Recognize the signs and symptoms of the deteriorating child
- Instigate appropriate intervention to prevent further deterioration
- Give BLS
- Summon expert help
- Assist in the administration of swift and efficient ALS.

Nurses can then carry out their vital role in the prevention of cardiopulmonary arrest in children and infants and increase their chances of recovery.

Nurses should seek sponsorship from their managers to attend paediatric ALS courses and ensure that they update their own professional knowledge and practice by attending their own hospital update courses.

Community-based staff should be able to provide training on paediatric BLS to the public, with midwives and health visitors providing this education to parents of the newborn. Various charities also exist, such as the Royal Life Saving Society, who have produced superb literature written for the general public, as well as providing voluntary trainers.

Finally, nurses who care for children must be aware of the painful emotional consequences of cardiorespiratory resuscitation attempts, and ensure that after these sad events

- The child's family is supported with sensitivity and compassion
- Staff are supported in structured reflection to ensure that learning can take place from all experiences, even the painful ones
- Emotions can be explored and all possible problems resolved.

In doing this, nurses will become more confident and competent practitioners in providing expert clinical care, as well as sensitive emotional care in the saddest and most distressing situations. They will then be able to help others, in particular the child's family, to begin to get through this desperate time.

REFERENCES

Advanced Life Support Group 1997 Advanced Paediatric Life Support: the practical approach, 2nd edn. BMJ Publishing Group, London, pp. 4–5

American Heart Association 1997 Paediatric advanced life support. American Heart Association, ch 1 pp. 1-1, ch 2 pp. 2-1

Benner P 1984 From novice to expert: excellence and power and clinical nursing practice. Addison-Wesley, Menlo Park

Bossaert L (ed.) 1998 European Resuscitation Council guidelines for resuscitation. Elsevier Science, Amsterdam

Connors P 1996 Should relatives be allowed in the resuscitation room? Nursing Standard 44:42–44

Johns C 1993 Professional supervision. Journal of Nursing Management 1:9–18

Resuscitation Council (UK) 1998 The 1998 resuscitation guidelines for use in the United Kingdom. Resuscitation Council (UK), London

Robson S 1998 The psychological effects of witnessing resuscitation on bereaved relatives. Lancet 352:614–618

United Kingdom Central Council for Nursing, Midwifery and Health Visiting (UKCC) 1992 Code of Professional Conduct. UKCC, London

Trauma resuscitation

Steve Rochester

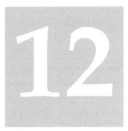

INTRODUCTION

Imagine trauma as a disease that can strike anyone at any time and has the ability to ignore who you are, where you work or what car you drive. It is stated in the advanced trauma life support (ATLS) manual (American College of Surgeons 1997) that trauma accounts for more deaths in the age range of 1–40 than any other condition. With this in mind, it is amazing that we do not do more to educate society in an attempt to reduce morbidity and mortality. It not only kills, it also maims, disables and disrupts peoples' lives both physically and psychologically.

Trauma resuscitation today owes much to courses such as the ATLS or Advanced Trauma Nursing Course (ATNC). The ATLS course originated from the United States of America, after an orthopaedic surgeon, Dr James Styner crashed his plane into woodland in Nebraska, USA, in February 1976. Unfortunately, his wife died and he and his children were injured in the crash. Following this disaster he and his colleagues set about attempting to improve resuscitation of the trauma patient. It was through Styner and his colleagues that the world learned how to deal with the trauma patient. Whether you love, hate or are indifferent to the variety of courses that are available to teach how to manage trauma, there is no escaping the fact that there is an identified need for such training and education. As long as trauma exists within our society we need to seek the best way or ways of managing it.

The governing body for trauma in the United Kingdom is the Royal College of Surgeons of England, which in turn takes its lead from the American College of Surgeons Committee on Trauma. These are separate and independent from the European Resuscitation Council and the Resuscitation Council (UK).

THE GOLDEN HOUR

Time in trauma resuscitation is vital to the outcome of the patient. The term 'the golden hour' (American College of Surgeons 1997) is used to convey the pressing need to instigate effective resuscitation. If a trauma occurs at 10.00 hours, but the patient does not arrive in the accident and emergency (A&E) department until 10.30 hours, only 30 min of the golden hour remain. Obviously, there will be occasions when the patient is trapped at the scene of the accident for a considerable time, and their golden hour may expire without hospitalization. In these situations it is probably more important to transport these patients as quickly as possible to the nearest appropriate hospital. Patients cannot be given definitive care while they remain at the scene.

Death in trauma occurs in a three-point distribution (the Trimodal Death Distribution, American College of Surgeons 1997):

1. The first point concerns those who will die at the scene because of massive disruption of organs such as the heart, brain or aorta. These people are unsavable.
2. The second point concerns patients who have an opportunity to survive if resuscitation is effected within the 'golden hour'.
3. The third point relates to patients who survived the initial insult, but will die on critical care units because of multi-organ dysfunction or sepsis.

How do injuries occur? 'Kinematics' is the process of assessing the incident and attempting to establish what motion and forces may have been involved (Hafen et al. 1996). This principle relates to Newton's first law of motion, which states that a body at rest will remain at rest, and a body in motion will remain in motion, unless acted on by an outside force. What this means to the trauma patient is that if they were involved in an incident involving a car that suddenly stops, e.g. crashes into a wall, their movements will have been acted upon by an external force, i.e. the wall. This change in energy and rapid deceleration force has the potential to cause profound injuries (ibid.); therefore, the ability to decelerate gradually in these situations will result in a better outcome for the patient.

The 'mechanism of injury' (Hafen et al. 1996) refers to how a patient is injured. It allows us to begin to piece together the nature of the incident and helps identify what may have happened to the patient at the time of the trauma. It is important with all trauma patients to understand the mechanism of injury. If we know how the trauma occurred then we may be able to anticipate what injuries they might have sustained and therefore have greater awareness of what treatment should be instigated. It must be remembered that mechanism of injury may result in blunt and/or penetrating trauma.

So what is meant by the mechanism of injury? Take the example of a road traffic accident (RTA). The receiving nurse in the A&E department will want accurate information about the patient and what happened at the accident scene. The A&E staff merely being told that they are receiving an RTA is not much help. The best people to provide appropriate information are the patients themselves or pre-hospital staff. What one needs to know is (Hafen *et al.* 1996):

- How many casualties there are
- What type of car the casualty was in
- The speed at which the accident occurred
- Were the occupants wearing seat belts, if they were not, were they ejected from the vehicle
- Did the car have airbags fitted and were they activated at the crash scene
- Was it a front, rear or lateral impact.

With that information you can now get on with the job at hand and resuscitate the patient. It must be noted that people involved in an RTA may have suffered both blunt trauma (seatbelt injury) and penetrating trauma (car's framework or outside factor, e.g. a fence post, penetrating their anatomy). It is therefore important to remember possible internal injuries and not attend only to open, visible wounds.

TRAUMA TEAMS

A trauma team should be readily available and be summoned to the A&E department by a hospital 'bleep' system. The composition of the team will depend upon what staff are employed within the hospital. A typical team for a District General Hospital will be the following members of staff:

- A&E consultant
- A&E senior house officer
- Specialist registrar
- A&E nursing staff (x 2–3)
- Anaesthetic specialist registrar
- Operating department assistant
- Orthopaedic specialist registrar
- General surgical specialist registrar
- Radiographer
- Resuscitation officer.

Their roles within the team will vary depending upon their levels of expertise.

The team members should be clearly identified (e.g. lead aprons marked 'nurse team leader', etc.) and the number of people in the resuscitation bay restricted to a minimum. Anyone wishing to observe the trauma call should be kept at a distance, allowing the team members space to work. All team members should adopt universal precautions (gloves, gowns, protective glasses/face shields) when treating a trauma patient to avoid possible risk of infection or contamination.

A first trauma call can be a frightening experience for the inexperienced nurse and the nurse team leader should look out for any 'stage fright' or inability to cope with the situation. Supervision and support may be required from more experienced nurses.

Trauma patients present with a wide variety and severity of symptoms so that it can be difficult to make junior staff appreciate how ill these patients may actually be. Patients may appear to be minimally injured even when they have sustained serious injuries. People tend to compensate for their injuries until they reach a point of no return, after which it becomes virtually impossible to resuscitate them. The compensatory mechanisms of the human body have two main functions: (1) maintaining cardiac output and blood pressure, and (2) restoring blood volume (Hafen *et al.* 1996).

Initially, the body is able to use its own defence mechanisms to maintain function, in most cases the patient may exhibit minimal or no signs of potential injury: this is compensatory shock (Porth 1994, Hafen *et al.* 1996). The initial fall in blood pressure is detected by the baroreceptors, leading to activation of the sympathetic nervous system. Adrenaline (epinephrine) and noradrenaline (norepinephrine) are released, causing peripheral vasoconstriction and an increased heart rate and the force at which the blood is expelled from the left ventricle (Porth 1994); this aids the body in compensating for any injury that has occurred. The release of adrenaline also has effects on the respiratory function of the patient, causing bronchodilation (to increase oxygenation), as well as affecting other body organs (see Box 12.1). Hypotension also stimulates the juxtaglomerular apparatus to

---

Box 12.1 Signs of compensatory/decompensatory shock

Compensatory mechanisms:
  Restlessness/anxiety
  Minimal tachycardia (very early sign of compensating)
  Normal/slightly decreased blood pressure
  Pale/cool skin
  Peripheral constriction of hands/feet (increased peripheral resistance)
Decompensatory mechanisms:
  Slow, shallow, irregular respiration
  Dilated pupils, reacting slowly
  Hypotension (systolic 90 mmHg or lower)
  Tachycardia (100–120 beats/min)
  Confusion
  Extreme pallor
  Cold extremities
  (Porth 1994, Hafen *et al.* 1996)

activate the renin–angiotensin mechanism resulting in vasoconstriction and fluid is shifted from the interstitial and intracellular spaces into the intravascular space to maintain blood pressure. The initial hypotension also causes feedback from the osmoreceptors resulting in the release of anti-diuretic hormone from the posterior pituitary. This has vasopressor effects, as well as reducing urinary volume in a further attempt to maintain blood pressure. If there is no stabilization of the injuries present, more blood will be shunted from the peripheries and less-vital organs to the vital organs, i.e. the heart, brain, lungs (ibid.). At this stage, the body is no longer able to function without intervention. Decompensatory shock sets in and the body requires external support to maintain equilibrium of the body systems. If stabilization of decompensatory shock does not occur multisystem organ damage, or irreversible shock will follow (Porth 1994, Hafen et al. 1996). The severe damage that results will cause death of an individual.

TRAUMA CENTRES

In the USA, trauma centres are an accepted part of the infrastructure in medicine, but in the UK this is not the case. The need for trauma centres in the UK was an issue raised by Adedeji & Driscoll (1996) but, to date, there has been no conclusive decision on the matter.

METHOD OF TREATMENT

All trauma patients are treated with the same method of approach. That method is to address the following aspects in the order shown:

A Airway maintenance with cervical spine protection
B Breathing and ventilation
C Circulation and haemorrhage
D Disability/neurological status
E Exposure/environmental control

The 'A,B,C,D,E' method (American College of Surgeons 1997) is a stan-dardized, practised approach which acts as a model for prioritizing the care of the patient. It may seem a very simplistic way to treat a patient and that is because it is. (Simple methods work!) The method works because an air-way problem will always kill a patient more quickly than a circulatory problem and if a trauma patient is approached in the above manner then injuries will be prioritized and dealt with accordingly. It is important when treating the trauma patient not to become distracted by something that may appear dramatic, but is not a life-threatening injury. Most pre-hospital staff are now trained to a high standard and will deliver the patient appropri-ately 'collared and backboarded' to the hospital. This is a means whereby a semi-rigid neck collar and a spinal immobilization board are used to maintain alignment of the spine and minimize any movement that could aggravate injury (American College of Surgeons 1997). If the mechanism of injury suggests that the patient may have a spinal injury, then it is safest to assume that one exists until it can be proven otherwise by clinical and radiological examination. Do not underestimate how frightening and uncomfortable it can be for trauma patients, especially children, to be strapped to a spinal board. They are unable to move, cold and often in pain. A simple explanation of what is happening, reassurance and physical contact, such as holding the patient's hand, and standing in their line of sight can reduce a patient's anxieties and fears and give great comfort.

A – airway with cervical spine control

The patient's airway can be assessed in a variety of ways but the most obvious is to accept that if they can talk to you they have a clear airway. However, if the patient presents in a state of unconsciousness the airway must be opened in a manner that does not introduce possible harm or exacerbate any spinal injuries. The manoeuvres to open the airway are jaw thrust or chin lift (American College of Surgeons 1997). Both of these are performed while the cervical spine is being immobilized. To achieve this either manual in-line immobilization (a member of staff physically holding the head and cervical spine in line) with or without a semi-rigid collar, or a semi-rigid collar and a head immobilization device should be employed.

If the airway does not improve with jaw thrust/chin lift and the oropharynx is free of secretions, blood or vomit, then it may be prudent to consider the use of an oral or nasopharyngeal airway (Advanced Life Support Course Subcommittee 1998), provided that there are no contraindications for their use, e.g. a basal skull fracture which prohibits anything being inserted nasally. A patient with a gag reflex will not readily tolerate an oropharyngeal airway (Hafen et al. 1996). All trauma patients should receive high flow (10–12 L/min) oxygen therapy via a mask with a reservoir that provides the highest inspired oxygen concentration possible, until their oxygen and ventilatory status has been assessed (Advanced Life Support Course Subcommittee 1998). Should the patient require tracheal intubation it should be performed by the most experienced anaesthetist available, while maintaining cervical spine immobilization. It may be helpful in this circumstance to undo the collar to allow greater opening of the mouth (Hafen et al. 1996, American College of Surgeons 1997). Because of the potential of cervical spine injury this situation calls for effective teamwork.

The cervical spine is deemed to be 'clear' once a cervical spine X-ray with clear visualization of vertebrae C7/T1 has been taken, or a computed tomography (CT) scan has been assessed by a senior doctor who is competent to make such decisions. If there is any doubt concerning the cervical spine then it must be assumed that an injury is still present.

B – breathing

Assessment of breathing will encompass the usual assessment of 'look, listen and feel' (Advanced Life Support Course Subcommittee 1998), but it is

Box 12.2 Factors that may inhibit respiration

Tension pneumothorax – a one-way valve effect that allows air into the pleural space but does not allow air to escape. Over a short period of time this will collapse the lung of the affected side (McSwain *et al.* 1990). This will shift the trachea and the heart, causing a twisting effect on the blood vessels and preventing blood from entering the heart, resulting in a backpressure that may be seen clinically in the neck veins, which may appear 'raised'. Eventually, the opposite lung will also collapse. A tension pneumothorax should be diagnosed clinically and not radiologically, i.e. observe for asymmetrical chest movement and tracheal deviation, hyperresonance will be present upon percussion, and there maybe diminished, even absent breath sounds (American College of Surgeons 1997).

Haemothorax – as the name suggests there is a collection of blood within the pleural space, possibly due to a tear from a blood vessel (McSwain *et al.* 1990). This condition will cause both ventilation and circulatory problems. An intravenous fluid challenge (normally 1 L of warmed Hartmann's solution) is given as a bolus and should be instigated prior to the insertion of the chest drain to compensate for the blood loss (ibid.).

Open pneumothorax (sometimes referred to as a sucking chest wound) – the initial management is to cover the wound with a dressing, which can be taped down on three sides to provide the effect of a 'flutter valve'. Upon inspiration, the dressing will prevent air from entering the thoracic cavity; as the patient exhales, the side which is not taped allows the air to exit (McSwain et al. 1990).

Flail chest – this is normally associated with multiple rib fractures. The ribs fracture in more than two places, resulting in a segment that appears to be free and acts against the unaffected ribs. This prevents normal respiration as there appears to be a floating chest wall with paradoxical movement (the flail segment is pulled inwards on inspiration while the ribs move outwards). The resulting pain inhibits respiration and therefore leads to a state of hypoxia (McSwain *et al.* 1990). It may mean that the patient, who may be awake and fully orientated, needs to be anaesthetized, intubated and ventilated to correct the hypoxic episode and allow the fractures time to heal (ibid.).

not sufficient merely to say that they are breathing or they are not breathing (apnoeic) (see Box 12.2). Factors to be considered are the mechanics of respiration, respiratory rate and pattern, plus investigations such as pulse oximetry and arterial blood gas analysis (American College of Surgeons 1997). This will then give a more comprehensive assessment of the patient's oxygenation and ventilatory status.

C – circulation

Assessment of the patient's circulatory status may be conducted by assessment of the factors in Box 12.3.

Any suspicion that the patient may be in shock requires a fluid challenge, after which the patient's condition should be reassessed. Intravenous access should be attempted by whatever route is achievable, ideally two large bore intravenous lines should be established i.e. a 14/16 gauge cannula, in each antecubital fossa (Evans 1990). Once intravenous access has been established, blood samples should be drawn for crossmatch and urea and electrolyte analysis. If it is not possible to gain peripheral access to a vein, then a venous cutdown may be performed at either the greater saphenous vein (ankle) or basilic vein (elbow). Central venous catheters can be associated with complications, such as a pneumothorax, inability to cannulate the vein and infection (Advanced life Support Subcommittee 1998), which may restrict their use. In addition, the patient may have a potential or actual cervical spine injury, which may restrict movement of the patient's head and neck for insertion of the catheters.

There is much debate over the best fluid of choice (crystalloid or colloid). Obviously, any patient who is bleeding requires blood, but it may not always be possible to supply this in the early stages of resuscitation. It must be remembered, however, that whatever fluid is administered it should be warmed to prevent further hypothermia. Intravenous fluids are stored at room temperature (25°C); if a patient is normothermic (37°C)

Box 12.3 Factors in the assessment of circulatory status

Level of consciousness – if the patient can communicate coherently, they must have an adequate blood volume and corresponding cerebral perfusion pressure (Skinner *et al.* 1991).

Capillary refill time – the normal refill time is < 2 s. It must be appreciated that conditions such as hypothermia or peripheral vasoconstriction caused by medications may increase the capillary refill time.

Blood pressure – a patient's blood pressure is not the sole indicator of shock. As stated in the ATLS provider manual (American College of Surgeons 1997), a trauma patient can lose between 15 and 30% of their circulating volume and still remain normotensive owing to initiation of compensatory mechanisms. Once they lose 50% or more they will become unconscious and deteriorate rapidly (Evans 1990).

Pulses – central and peripheral pulses should be assessed. If the peripheral pulses are absent and central pulses are weak, this may be indicative of decompensated shock.

Urinary output – if the patient is receiving aggressive fluid resuscitation then there should be some evidence of urinary output. A normal approximation of adequate urine output is 0.5 mL/kg/h.

administration of such fluid at the appropriate rate required may induce hypothermia. This is more marked when using blood or human albumin solution which is stored at a temperature of 4°C.

There are devices available which aid a trauma team by both warming fluids and providing pressure infusion simultaneously. If it is deemed that the patient is haemorrhaging, volume replacement is merely a means of buying time until surgical intervention can rectify the cause.

D – disability

Why disability? Simply because 'n' for neurological does not follow the alphabet, and as stated earlier, simple methods work. Assessment and management of head injuries should still follow the 'A, B, C,' pattern. Even if the patient presents with an obvious head injury do not let yourself or the team become distracted by it. Stick to the action plan.

If a debate arises about whether fluid should be given to this patient, because it might promote cerebral oedema, remember that a ruptured organ with uncontrolled haemorrhage will kill the patient more quickly than any head injury (American College of Surgeons 1997). The most appropriate course of action, therefore, would be to administer a fluid challenge and consult a neurosurgeon without delay.

It is imperative that the patient's blood pressure is maintained at a constant level. This is because the blood pressure makes up part of the equation of the cerebral perfusion pressure (CCP):

$$CCP = \text{blood pressure (BP)} - \text{intra cranial pressure (ICP)}$$

The importance of maintaining the CPP is not to be underestimated.

There are many anecdotal reports of patients with a head injury who are transferred to a neurosurgical centre and die on arrival due to obvious haemorrhage that has not been addressed. Dunn (1997) reported that 15% of patients transferred to the regional neurosurgical unit were hypotensive. This can also occur during intra-hospital transfer. The rush to get the patient to the CT suite can have the same disastrous consequences. Haemodynamically unstable patients should only leave the resuscitation room to go to the operating theatre.

Assessment of neurological injuries is based on a system called the Glasgow Coma Scale (GCS) (Teasdale & Jennett 1974). The GCS is a system that allows standardization in the assessment of patients with a head injury. The maximum score available is 15; the minimum score is 3 (see Box 12.4). The total is achieved by obtaining the best score from eye (E) plus motor (M) plus verbal (V) assessment.

Patients who have a Glasgow Coma Score of eight or less are deemed to be in coma. If this is the case, the patient will require intubation and ventilation. This is carried out with immobilization of the cervical spine, as described previously. The patient may be ventilated to maintain an arterial partial pressure of carbon dioxide ($PaCO_2$) level at an acceptable level (3.5–4.5 kPa) to prevent further cerebral haemorrhage. Carbon dioxide is a powerful vasodilator: as the $PaCO_2$ level rises it increases the risk of

Box 12.4 Glasgow Coma Scale. Teasdale & Jennet 1974, reproduced with permission of The Lancet Ltd.

Eye (E) – eye opening
Spontaneous	4
To speech	3
To pain	2
None	1

Motor (M) – best motor response
Obeys commands	6
Localizes pain	5
Normal flexion (withdrawal)	4
Abnormal flexion (decorticate)	3
Extension (decerebrate)	2
None (flaccid)	1

Verbal (V) – verbal response
Orientated	5
Confused conversation	4
Inappropriate words	3
Incomprehensible sounds	2
None	1

haemorrhage. Therefore, to prevent an increased risk of haemorrhage the patient's respiratory rate should be increased, thereby decreasing the level of carbon dioxide (Oh 1991).

E – evaluation

Having got to this stage, the patient should have had any life-threatening injuries dealt with accordingly. One can now evaluate and assess the patient as a whole, before moving onto the secondary survey. This will be the time to perform a 'log roll', i.e. rolling the patient while maintaining in-line immobilization of the cervical spine and spinal column (American College of Surgeons 1997), to examine the patient's back and perform a per rectal (PR) examination. Unless there is an indication to the contrary, the spinal board (if the patient is on one) may now be removed. Ensure at this stage that the patient is kept warm and that any analgesia, and anti-emetic, is administered. If the patient requires a blood transfusion ensure that the blood is obtained and carefully checked prior to administration.

The timing of necessary X-rays will vary from case to case but should not prevent resuscitation from occurring. An X-ray may have to be put on hold while a procedure such as an insertion of a chest drain is performed. If in doubt resuscitate first and take the films later. Other procedures such as 12–lead electrocardiogram (ECG) recordings and urinary catheterization may now be performed.

As the primary survey draws to a close and the secondary survey begins, remember to reassess and make frequent observations to ensure that the patient's clinical condition remains stable and is, hopefully, improving. The 'AMPLE' mnemonic is sometimes used to ascertain further history (American College of Surgeons 1997):

A – Allergies. Is the patient allergic to any substances or medications?
M – Medications. Does the patient take or use any drugs?
P – Past medical history.
L – Last food or drink. What and when did the patient last eat or drink?
E – Event. Can the patient remember anything about the incident?

SECONDARY SURVEY

This is a complete and thorough examination of the patient from head to foot to ensure that no wounds or fractures have been missed. Procedures such as minor suturing or back slab plasters can now be applied.

TRANSFER FOR DEFINITIVE CARE PROVISION

Once the patient has been fully resuscitated then they should be transported to the definitive care setting. This will require either intra- or inter-hospital transport to an intensive care unit (ICU), a ward or a specialist centre, e.g. a neurosurgical unit. There are many problems associated with transfer and, ideally, the most experienced staff should accompany the patient. Should there be deterioration in the patient's condition en route, the staff must be conversant with equipment and resuscitative procedures. The Intensive Care Society (1997) has made recommendations with regard to transporting critically ill patients. These include ensuring that the nursing staff who escort the patient, should be qualified to the English National Board (ENB) 100 or equivalent level. The standard of care and monitoring should be maintained at the same level as that within the ICU, operating theatre or A&E department.

The mode of transport, such as the use of a land ambulance or of a helicopter, is also determined by a number factors. The time scale is of considerable importance, but matters such as the availability of an appropriate helicopter and landing sites at both the transferring and receiving hospitals must be considered. In addition, space, weight and equipment restrictions may not lend themselves to air transfer. When transferring patients, as well as preparing them, it is important to prepare yourself, taking warm clothing – not only patients feel nauseous during transfer – remember anti-emetic, toilet, drink and you should consider money. Another important and often overlooked question is how are you, as the escorting nurse, going to get back to your hospital? It has been known for staff to become stranded a long way from home.

EQUIPMENT

What equipment an A&E department should have is a matter of local availability and preference. Ideally, there should be a dedicated room available for trauma patients 24 h a day. This would have the necessary equipment for resuscitation such as intubation and ventilation, possibly an anaesthetic machine, full patient monitoring, including invasive pressure monitoring, fluid warmers and pressure delivery systems, arterial blood gas analysis, X-ray facilities and lead aprons for the staff.

CARDIAC ARREST IN TRAUMA

This is normally the end result of problems such as hypoxia or massive haemorrhage. Cardiac arrest in trauma patients will normally have a poor prognosis, unless the aetiology is such that the problem can readily and easily be rectified. A recent study by Suominen *et al.* (1998) addressed overall survival rate in paediatric traumatic cardiac arrest. The study found that the survival rates remained low, irrespective of the mechanism of injury or initial cardiac arrest ECG rhythm.

MAJOR INCIDENTS

Everyone hopes that these will never occur, but they can and do strike at any place and time. The business of planning and preparation for the event is therefore crucial. Dress rehearsals although often criticised as being unrealistic, will always serve a useful purpose; even if they identify the smallest of problems they will have been worthwhile. Equipment and clothing locked in a cupboard year after year will become outdated and therefore unsuited to requirements when needed.

CRITICAL INCIDENT DEBRIEFING

Following any incident there should be an attempt to review the trauma call. This will serve two purposes: critical review of the event and clinical procedures (this will identify strengths and weaknesses) and education of staff.

Trauma life support is very stressful for patients, staff and relatives. Quite apart from the professional demands for advanced knowledge and skill, there is also emotional stress. Inexperienced staff may find this very difficult and will require support, teaching and encouragement to build their confidence and enable them to deal with these dramatic and distressing events.

REHABILITATION

Once the initial incident has passed, the task of healing begins both physically and psychologically. Much time and money will be invested in an attempt to return the patient to their normal lifestyle, so it is important that no area is missed. Trauma is often seen as the sole remit of the trauma team but other staff, such as physiotherapists, occupational therapists and counsellors, will help in the lengthy rehabilitation process.

PREVENTION AND EDUCATION

What are we doing to reduce the impact of trauma upon society? Various improvements have been made by car manufacturers, road builders, etc., but we are still a long way from our goal. If we cannot prevent trauma then we should prepare ourselves to deal with it effectively. We must look back to where it all started with Dr Styner in 1976:

'When I can provide better care in the field with limited resources than that my children and I received at the primary care facility, there is something wrong with the system and the system has to be changed.'

(Styner 1976)

Education of all grades of staff involved with trauma, both pre-hospital and in hospital, is the only way to ensure appropriate treatment is delivered to our patients.

CONCLUSION

Trauma is a disease of such epidemic levels that it is truly frightening. As Doelp (1993) states:

'eight-thousand children a year die as a result of accidents in the United States of America. For each child that dies, one-hundred more are injured.'

I was fortunate enough undertake my Paediatric advanced life support (PALS) provider course at Children's Hospital National Medical Center in Washington DC, USA, a level 1 trauma centre. It was this experience that made me change my working practices and my way of thinking, not only about paediatric resuscitation, but about the way in which we must spread the message about this disease that lies in wait, ready to attack its next unsuspecting victim. It struck me during the course that there is very little taught about trauma resuscitation throughout a nurse's training. With the exception of an A&E placement, a student nurse, or for that matter a qualified nurse, has little or no education and training about how to deal with trauma. Although the existence of courses such as the ATLS or ATNC have to some degree addressed this issue for qualified nurses, it is still generally true that a disease that kills and maims the young goes virtually unnoticed throughout most nurses' training; it is hoped that this chapter goes some way towards addressing this deficit. Remember, if trauma can affect a princess and a president, it can affect any one of us, at anytime.

REFERENCES

Adedeji O A, Driscoll P A 1996 The Trauma Team – a system of initial care. Postgraduate Medical Journal 72(852):587–593
Advanced Life Support Subcommittee 1998 Advanced life support course provider manual, 3rd edn. Resuscitation Council UK, London

American College of Surgeons 1997 Advanced trauma life support for doctors, 1st impression. American College of Surgeons, Chicago

Doelp A 1989 In the blink of a eye. Prentice Hall, Englewood Cliffs

Dunn L T 1997 Secondary insults during the interhospital transfer of head-injured patients: an audit of transfers in the Mersey region. Injury 287:427–431

Evans T R (ed.) 1990 ABC of resuscitation. British Medical Journal, Cambridge

Hafen B Q, Karren K J, Misovich J J 1996 Prehospital emergency care, 5th edn. Prentice Hall, Englewood Cliffs

Intensive Care Society 1997 Guidelines for the transport of the critically ill patient. The Intensive Care Society, London

McSwain N E, Butman A M, McConnell W K, Vomacka R W (eds) 1990 Prehospital trauma life support manual, 2nd edn. Emergency Training, Akron

Oh T E 1991 Intensive care manual, 3rd edn. Butterworth, Sydney

Porth C M 1994 Pathophysiology: concepts of altered health states, 4th edn. J B Lippincott, Philadelphia

Skinner D, Driscoll P, Earlam R (eds) 1991 ABC of major trauma. British Medical Journal, London

Styner J 1976 Cited in: American College of Surgeons 1997, ch 1

Suominen P, Rasanen J, Kivioja A 1998 Efficacy of cardiopulmonary resuscitation in pulseless paediatric trauma patients. Resuscitation 36(1):9–13

Teasdale G, Jennett B 1974 Assessment of coma and impaired consciousness: a practical scale. Lancet ii:81–84

Resuscitation in the community

Barbara Plumb

INTRODUCTION

Nurses who work in the community may have to resuscitate in the home, the community hospital or clinic, the general practitioner (GP) surgery, the dental practice, the school or college, or perhaps the street. The victim may be of any age, from the neonate to the very elderly. The public has a right to expect that nurses should be able to provide basic life support (BLS) even in an 'off-duty' situation (UKCC 1992 Code of Conduct, clauses 1, 2 and 3). However, dealing with cardiorespiratory arrest in the out-of-hospital setting, perhaps without colleague support or equipment can be a daunting prospect, even for the most experienced nurse. BLS and advanced life support (ALS) procedures are discussed in chapters 6 and 7, respectively, and will not be described in detail here. In this chapter, I discuss some of the problems that nurses may encounter in a variety of community contexts and also look at means of problem solving for the nurse working in these settings. Anaphylaxis is included in the section on resuscitation in GP surgeries. This is purely for convenience since it can occur in any health-care setting. The importance of summoning assistance and instigating life support is emphasized throughout, for it remains the mainstay of resuscitation in all community contexts, just as it is within the hospital setting.

The outcome in out-of-hospital resuscitation remains poor (see chapter 8) and nurses have a duty to ensure that everything possible is done to save a life. In order to do so, community nurses must ensure that they have and maintain the necessary skills and knowledge to resuscitate competently. Nurses are responsible for their own knowledge base for practice and should be able to show evidence of regular updating of BLS skills as part of their professional accountability (UKCC 1992). Community nurses should have skills in both adult and paediatric resuscitation which should be updated at regular intervals. As health care professionals they should also ensure that the necessary equipment is provided to enable them to carry

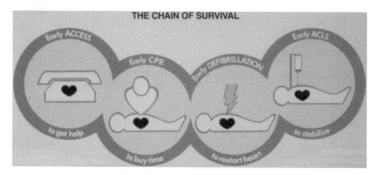

Fig. 13.1 The Chain of Survival. Reproduced with the permission of Laerdal Medical Ltd, Orpington, UK.

out their role in resuscitation. Although there is little evidence to suggest risk to the rescuer from the performance of mouth-to-mouth (Resuscitation Council (UK) 1998, chapter 3) most agencies suggest the use of a pocket mask or face shield, if available. Nurses should be prepared to take an active role in the purchase of emergency equipment and advising on emergency procedures in their working environment to ensure the safety of patients and staff at all times.

Risk assessment is the key issue in managing cardiopulmonary arrest in the community. It should be carried out for all areas in which patient care is carried out and plans or protocols should be prepared to ensure that a swift, organized, controlled and carefully considered response can be made in the event of a cardiorespiratory arrest. All nurses in all settings should be aware of the importance of the 'Chain of Survival' (Fig. 13.1). This model portrays the sequence of events required for a positive outcome from cardiopulmonary arrest both in and out of hospital.

GP SURGERIES

As general practice changes and primary care groups are formed, large out-of-hours cooperatives are emerging. GPs are becoming more aware of their role in the emergency situation (Barton & Wilson 1997, Bossaert 1998, pp 169–204). Automated external defibrillators (AEDs) are becoming more common in the surgery setting and resuscitation training needs are being identified (Heslitz *et al.* 1998, Weston 1998).

Some procedures performed in family planning clinics (e.g. the fitting of a coil) carry an increased risk of cardiopulmonary collapse, so equipment should be available and staff fully trained. In the general practice surgery setting, there may be more equipment available and, usually, other health-care professionals to assist. Support staff, such as receptionists, secretaries and cleaners, are also employed and may be the first people to find the collapsed victim. It is therefore essential that all medical, nursing and support staff should be trained regularly in the use of emergency procedures and

BLS. Practice nurses may be required to take responsibility for training staff in emergency procedures. This should involve training all staff in BLS, activation of an internal emergency call system and ensuring that reception staff know how to activate the external emergency (999) system. (The simplest and cheapest internal call system I have ever encountered is a sports whistle on a string hanging behind every door.)

Staff should also be familiar with the location of any emergency equipment and understand their role in supporting relatives and dealing with other patients/clients. A small surgery may need to be cleared of patients, while in larger practices they may remain unaware of what is going on in another part of the building. These decisions should be made in advance as part of the local protocol and each member of staff should know what their responsibilities are and how to carry them out. Ideally, nursing staff who are required to train others, should themselves have successfully completed the relevant courses in both adult and paediatric resuscitation provided by the Resuscitation Council (UK).

Health Centres and Surgeries are often situated in buildings that are old and were not purpose built. Inevitably, they may have a number of areas where, in the event of the sudden collapse of a patient, access and resuscitation would be difficult. Emergency procedures should be worked out in advance, so that staff are aware of local problems and know how best to proceed. Furniture that obstructs access should be removed and access to the building by emergency vehicles should also be considered.

Nurses carrying out procedures where anaphylaxis is a risk should have relevant emergency equipment and drugs available to them, such as adrenaline (Resuscitation Council (UK) 1998, chapter 11). The community nurse or health visitor may be involved in resuscitation within the practice setting and, if so, should be familiar with equipment and the procedure for getting help. If running an immunization session, adrenaline (epinephrine) 1:1000 should be available and should be given immediately if anaphylaxis occurs (Chamberlain *et al.* 1998, Resuscitation Council (UK) 1998, chapter 11); nurses whose practice includes immunization should be aware of its nature, pathogenesis and treatment.

Anaphylaxis

This is an exaggerated response of a previously sensitized individual to foreign allergenic material. It is an immediate hypersensitivity reaction caused most commonly by insect bites, certain foods, blood products and drugs.

Pathogenesis

Anaphylaxis is mediated by IgE antibodies, which cause histamine and other vasoactive mediators to be released from mast cells and basophils, producing respiratory, circulatory, cutaneous and gastro-intestinal effects. Increased vascular permeability and peripheral vasodilatation reduce venous return and cardiac output: sudden collapse and death can result.

Anaphylactoid reactions present in a similar manner, but there is no previous sensitization and IgE is not involved. The treatment is the same.

Diagnosis

This is based on:

- A feeling of faintness or impending doom (aura)
- Flushing
- An itchy rash, usually urticaria or erythema
- Facial swelling (angioedema) extending to the upper airway
- Bronchoconstriction
- Vomiting or diarrhoea
- Hypovolaemia and cardiovascular collapse associated with vasodilatation and an increase in vascular permeability

Resuscitation

The airway should be opened and maintained with the administration of 100% oxygen when available. If stridor, wheeze, respiratory distress or clinical signs of shock are present, 0.5 mL of adrenaline 1:1000 (500 μg) should be given intramuscularly (IM) immediately and repeated after 5 min if no clinical improvement is observed. This dose may need to be repeated at intervals to maintain the improvement thereafter.

Where there is profound shock, judged to be immediately life-threatening, cardiopulmonary resuscitation (CPR) should be commenced and 3–5 mL (300–500 μg) 1:10 000 adrenaline given slowly IV. This can then be repeated at 5 min if there is no clinical improvement. CPR or ALS should continue if required.

An antihistamine (e.g. chlorpheniramine 10–20 mg) can also be given by slow intravenous (IV) or IM injection. After severe attacks, hydrocortisone (as sodium succinate) may help to avert later sequelae. The adult dose is 100–500 mg by slow IV or IM injection.

Should severe hypotension not respond rapidly to drug therapy, fluids may be infused and colloids are recommended. One to two units may be required.

Equipment available within the surgery setting is variable and may be kept in a number of separate areas. Many surgeries have oxygen and suction available, and some have defibrillators and emergency airway and drug packs, as well as electrocardiogram (ECG) machines. Evidence encouraging the use of AEDs (Bossaert 1998, pp 118–126; Fig. 13.2) has convinced some GPs to invest in a defibrillator that can be used by multidisciplinary members of the team. If such equipment is available, procedures for BLS and the early use of defibrillation must be set up and regularly rehearsed (Bossaert et al. 1997; Fig. 13.1). After suitable training, the AED can be used by nurses and other staff who have the appropriate BLS skills (Resuscitation Council (UK) 1998, chapter 7). As with all resuscitation skills, AED training needs to be updated every 6–12 months. The most important factors in saving patients who suffer a cardiopulmonary arrest in Health Clinics and GP Surgeries are diagnosis of the arrest, the instigation of BLS, calling an ambulance and early defibrillation if available, so that the first links in the Chain of Survival are put into place and the patient's chance of survival is increased.

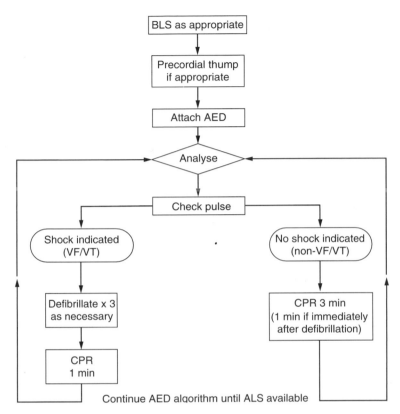

Cardiac arrest

BLS as appropriate

Precordial thump
if appropriate

Attach AED

Analyse

Check pulse

Shock indicated
(VF/VT)

No shock indicated
(non-VF/VT)

Defibrillate x 3
as necessary

CPR 3 min
(1 min if immediately
after defibrillation)

CPR
1 min

Continue AED algorithm until ALS available

Fig. 13.2 Automated external defibrillator (AED) algorithm.

THE HOME

Community nursing staff may be involved in a resuscitation attempt while visiting a patient at home, although not necessarily involving the patient they came in to see. This will involve them in BLS as a 'first responder' (see chapter 6), ideally using a pocket-mask or face-shield. CPR at home may be made difficult if a bedridden or heavy patient requires BLS on a non-hospital bed. Moving the patient to the floor may be difficult for the lone rescuer. A compromise arrangement using a breadboard or tray under the shoulders may improve the effectiveness of CPR. (A mobile telephone can be very useful in this situation.)

Factors such as having to unlock doors to allow entry for the paramedics or dealing with upset relatives make CPR in this setting more difficult for the single nurse. In such situations the nurse should always perform BLS until further help arrives (Handley *et al.* 1997, see also chapter 6).

It may not be appropriate to commence CPR on all patients and 'do not resuscitate' (DNR) policy guidelines may need to be discussed with the patient, their family and the GP (Resuscitation Council (UK) 1993). These discussions should have taken place in advance of any event but if there is any doubt the nurse has a duty to commence CPR and summon help.

COMMUNITY HOSPITALS

Community hospitals vary in size and some may have a defibrillator available. More community hospitals are perceiving the wisdom of buying AEDs that can be used by nursing staff. Oxygen and suction will normally be available as well as pocket-masks, bag-valve masks (BVM) and oropharyngeal airways, so staff need to be proficient in their use. (Resuscitation Council (UK) 1998, chapter 5).

Colleague support is usual, although the emergency (999) service will need to be activated because, in the event of successful resuscitation, it is likely that the patient will need to be transferred to a more suitable hospital for post-resuscitation care. It should be remembered that resuscitation is not necessarily appropriate for all patients in a community hospital, since many patients may be approaching the natural end of their lives or suffering from advanced pathologies which would render resuscitation both futile and unkind (see chapter 2 on the Ethical Aspects of Resuscitation). 'Do Not Resuscitate' (DNR) policies should be in place (Resuscitation Council (UK) 1993, National Council for Hospice and Specialist Palliative Care 1997, Bossaert 1998, pp 205–217) in these cases. Resuscitation status should be decided on an individual basis after open discussion involving the patient, when possible, and the family should be fully informed of the decision made and its rationales (see chapter 3). Nurses working in these areas should ensure that the subject of resuscitation is explored with patients as part of the nursing assessment. The patient's wishes should be discussed so that they can be offered the dignity of making their own decision. Their wishes should be recorded and communicated to the other professions involved in the patient's care.

Risk assessment in advance is important because there are often areas such as the physiotherapy gym or hydrotherapy pool in which, if a patient requiring resuscitation collapses, staff would face extra difficulties. Regular CPR training should be carried out (Wynne 1987) and staff debriefing needs to be available. Scenario practice helps staff to understand their roles and gives insight into local contextual problems. Action cards may help staff to be familiar with their roles in response to a resuscitation emergency. (Tilsted & Reid 1997). Consideration may need to be given to the use of the laryngeal mask airway as an airway management tool in community hospitals, if a skilled intubator is not readily available (Baskett 1994; see chapter 9). Adjuncts for improving chest compression are now available and can be used as a training aid or to improve effective compressions during a cardiac arrest. Specific training requirements may need to be addressed such as:

- Resuscitation of the pregnant woman (Resuscitation Council (UK) 1998, chapter 11)
- Procedures for choking in units for the mentally ill
- Adaptations for dealing with patients with physical disabilities
- Resuscitation techniques for the patient who has had a laryngectomy
- Paediatric resuscitation (ILCOR 1998; see chapter 11).

CARE HOMES

Patients in nursing or residential homes are now considered candidates for resuscitation (Resuscitation Council (UK) 1998, chapter 16). A large number of healthcare assistants provide care in these homes and they require regular training. Usually, BLS is commenced and the emergency (999) services called. Pocket-masks or face-shields should be available and some nursing homes may have BVMs, oxygen and suction to assist in airway management. It is useful to have practice CPR scenarios, which include role-play so that training needs, as well as practical problems, can be identified.

DNR policies should be in place (Bossaert 1998), and decisions should be made following discussion with the patient if possible, or by the GP and care staff. The decision should be discussed with the family but it should be remembered that they have no legal right to give or withhold permission for treatment (see chapter 3). Nurses should attempt to ascertain during the assessment process, what the patient's wishes are with regard to their own resuscitation. This indicates respect for the patient's dignity and autonomy and enables the nurse to take on the role of advocate. The patient's wishes should be recorded and communicated to other staff involved in the patient's care.

SCHOOL NURSES

School nurses need to be fully trained in both adult and paediatric BLS (ILCOR 1998). They need to be fully prepared to respond to emergencies such as anaphylaxis (see above) when carrying out immunization sessions, and may be called upon to assist in the event of accidents involving staff or pupils.

DENTAL SURGERIES

The Poswillo Report (1991) (Mason 1991) set a standard that was nationally accepted for the establishment of resuscitation procedures and equipment within the dental surgery. Two of the report's recommendations are:

- Every member of the dental team should be trained in resuscitation and training should be a team activity
- Resuscitation procedures should be regularly practised in the surgery under simulated conditions.

Box 13.1 HEARTSTART SCHEMES (BRITISH HEART FOUNDATION)

- Crewe Heartstart Dental Team Beat
- Cornwall Heartrace Dentist Scheme
- Halton and Chester Heartstart Dental Team Beat
- Kent Heartstart Dental
- Liverpool Heartstart Dental Team Beat
- Macclesfield Dental Team Beat
- Sefton Dental Team Beat
- St Helens and Knowlsley Dental Team Beat
- Wirral Dental Team Beat.

These recommendations have led to dental practices organizing regular sessions to update staff resuscitation skills using national health service (NHS) resuscitation officers, paramedic trainers and voluntary aid society trainers (Red Cross, St John and St Andrew Ambulance) or in some cases setting up their own heartstart training (see Box 13.1).

As CPR skills improved, concerns were expressed both in this country and elsewhere about the number of drugs kept, but very rarely used, in dental surgeries in accordance with the Poswillo Guidelines. An article by McCarthy (1993) starts with the introduction:

'Medical preparedness in Dentistry has become over-complicated: over-preparation without experience can lead to treatment skills that are not frequently applied to wither from disuse.'

This article, together with the reduction in the use of General Anaesthesia in Dental Surgeries, has instigated a review to update the Poswillo Report (1991). It is now recommended that dentists should have a working knowledge of

- CPR
- Heimlich manoeuvre
- Airway assessment (airway patency manoeuvre)
- Treatment of vomiting or airway foreign body (emesis/foreign body manoeuvre)
- Diagnosis and treatment of anaphylaxis
- Positive pressure ventilation
- Recognition and emergency treatment of common risk diseases such as angina pectoris, acute myocardial infarction and cerebrovascular accident.

Dental surgery settings need to be risk assessed for problem areas and emergency procedures need to be practised; buzzer or whistle emergency call systems need to be developed. A procedure for coping with patients waiting and arriving at the surgery must be considered. This may require an answer-phone message or a sign for the surgery door to cancel patients and these should be prepared in advance. A number of dentists and dental nurses now attend ALS courses run by the Resuscitation Council (UK) to ensure that emergency care in their surgeries is efficient, professional and competent.

GENERAL POINTS

Resuscitation in the nonacute (community) setting happens less frequently than in the acute hospital setting. When it does occur, the pressure on staff to cope with an unexpected immediate emergency causes increased stress for all involved. The victim is swiftly removed by the ambulance crew and, within a few minutes, it can appear as if nothing has happened. It is not easy to continue with the day's work after the resuscitation of a patient and all staff involved may be upset by what has happened. Nurses have more experience than most in dealing with death (see chapter 4) and it may fall upon the nursing staff to offer support to others. If a child was resuscitated, the grief and anxiety this causes may be extreme and necessitate the closure of the clinic or surgery for the rest of that day as staff may be unable to cope. Debriefing in these situations is very important so that staff can be encouraged to express and share their feelings. They may need help to accept what happened to come to terms with the drama of resuscitation. Reflection on the event can bring to light any procedural problems and help inexperienced staff to cope with such emergencies.

The nurse may have to contact the next of kin and inform them about what has happened and this can be very distressing (see chapter 5). Ideally, a nurse would carry out this sad task but, when developing roles within protocols, this should not be forgotten and should be allocated according to local staff availability.

CPR scenarios should be practised on a regular basis to keep skills updated (Wynne 1987). Action cards may be of use in GP or dental surgeries so that office staff and receptionists know their role. Call systems such as bell signals, whistles and code words over the intercom should be agreed and always acted upon. Risk assessment of all areas frequented by patients should be carried out to evaluate the best action. All emergency equipment should be checked regularly and all staff should be familiar with its location. Consideration should be given to improving outcome for patients by the use of the AED. Practical training in the use of the AED and airway management skills must be practised regularly. Local knowledge is useful, e.g. many dental practices link with general practices or health centres that may have a defibrillator available. The emergency (999) system activates immediate access to the emergency services. Many NHS ambulance trusts now provide telephone advice and this advice can be used in the resuscitation (McNaughton & Wyatt 1997).

Nurses may be involved in community resuscitation training programmes such as the 'Heartstart' scheme, coordinated nationally by the British Heart Foundation. They may also be involved with voluntary aid societies (such as the Red Cross or St John Ambulance) either in a training role or using their skills as part of volunteer medical teams at public events (Kerr & Parke 1999, Russel et al. 1999). Since 1998, appropriately trained nurses may become full members of the British Association of Immediate Care Schemes (BASICS).

OTHER CONSIDERATIONS

The nurse needs to be aware of ever-increasing sophistication in cardiac and resuscitative care.

The implantable cardioverter defibrillator (ICD) does not preclude the possibility of cardiac arrest. Patients with implantable defibrillators may present to the nurse who needs to be aware that there is no risk to the resuscitator if the defibrillator is activated. The presence of the ICD should not in any way alter the application of normal resuscitation procedures. External defibrillation even using an AED should be instigated if the dysrhythmia is appropriate (Calle & Buylaert 1998).

The CPR Plus is an adjunct that can improve the efficiency both of training and actual CPR skills. CPR Plus removes the hands from the patient's chest wall and makes precise and accurate chest compressions possible. A gauge enables compression depth to be assessed and guides the rescuer in a more accurate rate and rhythm.

The ambu cardio pump is a device that is used to achieve active compression–decompression in CPR (ACD-CPR). It has been suggested that ACD-CPR has been shown to improve blood circulation and allow more control over compression–decompression and rate and rhythm. However, different chest geometries have been shown to influence the effectiveness of the device and need to be considered when using it. The efficacy of this device has yet to be fully proven (Kern et al. 1996, Haid et al. 1997).

CONCLUSION

Innovations in resuscitation in the field of pre-hospital care continue to develop (Weston 1998) and the challenge of responding to these developments must be accepted by nurses as part of the primary health care team. The role of the nurse in community resuscitation is still evolving: providing skilled and compassionate care in the community setting is part of that role. The wide variety of contexts and locations in which nurses may be called upon to put into practice their BLS or ALS skills, create a constant need for regular and repeated training. It is essential that community nurses have the skills and knowledge to respond professionally in the event of the sudden collapse of patients, staff or passers by. The key points of this chapter are summarized in Box 13.2.

Box 13.2 KEY POINTS

- Early defibrillation has been shown to improve the chances of survival in the pre-hospital setting (Bossaert *et al.* 1997, Bossaert 1998).
- The introduction of AEDs means that nurses can potentially play a greater role when the need for resuscitation in the community occurs.
- In your working environment, you should be aware of what resuscitation equipment is available, where it is kept and how to use it.
- Your skills in BLS should be regularly updated to maintain professional competence.
- Emergency call systems and protocols, adapted to the local context, should be worked out in advance and regularly rehearsed.
- All staff in health care environments should be able to carry out BLS and be familiar with emergency call systems and protocols.
- Debriefing should be carried out after any serious emergency in order to adapt systems and protocols as necessary and to support staff who may be distressed.
- The 'Chain of Survival' is fundamental to survival in out-of-hospital resuscitation attempts, i.e. early access, early BLS, early defibrillation and early ALS.

REFERENCES

Barton P, Wilson P 1997 Emergencies in the community: general practitioners confidence levels and learning needs. A confidential survey. Pre-hospital Immediate Care 1:189–193

Baskett P 1994 Multicentre trial (coordinator Baskett P J F). The use of the laryngeal mask airway by nurses during cardio-pulmonary resuscitation. Anaesthesia 49:3–7

Bossaert L (ed.) 1998 European Resuscitation Council guidelines for resuscitation. Elsevier Science, Amsterdam

Bossaert L, Callanam V, Cummins R 1997 Early defibrillation. Resuscitation 34:113–114

Calle P, Buylaert W 1998 When an AED meets an ICD. Resuscitation 38:77–183

Chamberlain D, Ward M *et al.* 1998 The emergency treatment of anaphylactic reaction. For a project team of the Resuscitation Council (UK). Resuscitation Council UK

Haid C, Rabl W, Baubin M 1997 Active compression–decompression resuscitation: the influence of different chest geometries on the force transmission. Resuscitation 35:83–85

Handley A, Becker L, Allen M, van Dienth A, Montgomery W 1997 Single rescuer adult basic life support. An advisory statement by the basic life support working group of the International Liaison Committee on Resuscitation. Resuscitation 34:101–107

Heslitz J, Bang A, Axelsson A, Graves J, Lindquist J 1998 Experience with the use of automated external defibrillators in out of hospital arrest. Resuscitation 37:3–7

International Liaison Committee on Resuscitation 1998 Paediatric working group advisory statement. In: Bossaert L (ed.) European Resuscitation Council Guidelines for Resuscitation 1998. Elsevier (for the European Resuscitation Council), Amsterdam

Kern K, Figge C *et al.* 1996 Active compression/decompression versus standard cardiopulmonary resuscitation: a porcine model: no improvement in outcome. American Heart Journal 132/6:1156–1162

Kerr G, Parke T 1999 Providing 'T' in the part of pre-hospital care at a major crowd event. Pre-hospital Immediate Care 3:11–13

Mason D 1991 Statement from the President of the GDC. British Dental Journal January:47

McCarthy F 1993 Emergency drugs and devices–less or more? California Dental Association Journal February:19–25

McNaughton G W, Wyatt J P 1997 Telephone guided CPR–it's good to talk! Pre-hospital Immediate Care 1(2):71–72

National Council for Hospice and Specialist Palliative Care Services Joint Working Party 1997 Ethical decision making in palliative care: cardiopulmonary resuscitation CPR for people who are terminally ill. National Council for Hospice and Specialist Palliative Care Services, London

Poswillo D E 1991 Poswillo Report. Principle recommendations of the report. British Dental Journal 19:1–91 (General anaesthesia, sedation and resuscitation in dentistry. Report of expert working party. Department of Health, London)

Resuscitation Council (UK) 1993 Decisions relating to cardio-pulmonary resuscitation. A statement from the BMA and RCN in association with the Resuscitation Council (UK). British Medical Journal March

Resuscitation Council (UK) 1998 Advanced Life Support Course sub-committee of the Resuscitation Council (UK) (eds) Advanced Life Support Course – Provider Manual, 3rd edn. Resuscitation Council (UK), London

Russel R, Hodgetts T, Castle N 1999 Medical support to an organized race. Pre-hospital Immediate Care 3: 5–10

Tilsted J, Reid J 1997 Using action cards to improve resuscitation response. Nursing Standard 11(16):42–44

United Kingdom Central Council for Nursing, Midwifery and Health Visiting 1992 Code of professional conduct, 3rd edn. UKCC, London

Weston C 1998 Development of resuscitation after pre-hospital cardiac arrest. Pre-hospital Immediate Care 2(2):90–94.

Wynne G 1987 Inability of trained nurses to perform basic life support. British Medical Journal 294:1198–1199

Index

Index

*Note abbreviations used in subheadings: AEDs = automatic external defibrillators;
AICDS = automatic internal cardioverter defibrillators; ALS = advanced life support;
BLS = basic life support; EMD = electromechanical dissociation; PEA = pulseless electrical
activity; VF = ventricular fibrillation; VT = ventricular tachy-arrhythmias.*